DATE DUE

AUG 5 1986			

DEMCO 38-297

Gynaecological Oncology

Edited by
C. Paul Morrow and George E. Smart

With 75 Figures and 110 Tables

Springer-Verlag
Berlin Heidelberg New York Tokyo

C. Paul Morrow, MD
Department of Gynecologic Oncology
UCLA School of Medicine
Los Angeles
California, USA

George E. Smart, FRCOG, FRCSE
Department of Obstetrics and Gynaecology
University of Edinburgh
Edinburgh, Scotland, UK

ISBN 3-540-15775-1 Springer-Verlag Berlin Heidelberg New York Tokyo
ISBN 0-387-15775-1 Springer-Verlag New York Heidelberg Berlin Tokyo

Library of Congress Cataloging-in-Publication Data
Main entry under title:
Gynaecological oncology
Includes bibliographies and index.
1. Generative organs, Female – Cancer. I. Morrow, C. Paul, 1935– . II. Smart,
George E., 1935– . [DNLM: 1. Genital Neoplasms, Female. WP 145 G997]
RC280.G5G86 1985 616.99'265 85-17253
ISBN 0-387-15775-1 (U.S.)

Phototypesetting by Computerized Typesetting Services Ltd, North Finchley,
London. Printed by Henry Ling Limited, The Dorset Press, Dorchester

2128/3916-543210

To Jean and Margaret

Preface

This collection of papers on different aspects of gynaecological oncology is taken from the proceedings of the Second International Conference on Gynaecological Cancer held in Edinburgh in September 1983. An attempt has been made to include topical material of interest and importance to all gynaecologists, both with and without specific oncological experience, and it is confidently expected that radiotherapists and general surgeons will also find much of value within these pages.

Much of the material has been updated prior to its transfer to the printers, and authors have tried where possible to provide workable rather than tiresomely comprehensive bibliographies.

Our sincerest thanks are directed to our other colleagues on the Organising Committee, namely Professors J. Carmichael, W. Duncan and J. F. Smyth and Doctors I. Duncan, J. R. B. Livingstone, R. H. Nalick, T. J. O'Brien and E. Petrilli for their invaluable assistance on both sides of the Atlantic with the organisation of the above conference, to Dr. R. H. Kerr-Wilson for his help with, and sometimes translation of, the original proofs, and to our constantly overworked and uncomplaining secretaries Joann Little and Mary Hall.

Los Angeles and Edinburgh
1985

Paul Morrow
George Smart

Contents

SECTION III: Endometrium

SECTION IV: Ovary

Contributors

H. Advani, MD
Department of Pathology, Walter Reed Army Medical Center,
Washington DC 20307, USA

G. M. Awais, MD, FRCS(C), FACOG, FACS
Department of Gynecology, Cleveland Clinic Foundation,
Cleveland, Ohio, USA

V. Barley, DPhil, DMRT
Department of Radiotherapy, University of Bristol, Bristol,
England, UK

D. Barnhill, MD
Department of Obstetrics and Gynecology, Uniformed Services
University of Health Sciences, Bethesda, Maryland 20814, USA

M. S. Baylis, MB, MRCOG
Tenovus Institute for Cancer Research, Welsh National School of
Medicine, Heath Park, Cardiff CF4 4XX, Wales, UK

J. S. Berek, MD
Division of Gynecologic Oncology, UCLA School of Medicine,
Center for Ovarian Cancer, Johnsson Comprehensive Cancer
Care Center, Los Angeles, California 90024, USA

A. E. Bogden, PhD
Department of Medicine, E. G. & G. Mason Research Institute,
Worcester, MA 011608, USA

J. Bonte, MD
Department of Gynaecology, Academisch Ziekenhuis,
3000 Leuven, Sint-Rafael, Kapuclijnenvoer 33, Belgium

P. Brzozowski, MD
Department of Obstetrics and Gynecology, Uniformed Services
University of Health Sciences, Bethesda, Maryland 20814, USA

B. Bundy
COG Statistical Office, Buffalo, New York, USA

M. O. Burrell, MD
Department of Gynecology, St Joseph's Hospital, Atlanta,
Georgia, USA

J. A. Carmichael, MD
Department of Obstetrics and Gynecology, Queens University,
Kingston, Ontario, Canada

L. F. Carson, MD
Department of Obstetrics and Gynecology, University of
Minnesota Medical School, 420 Delaware Street Southeast,
Minneapolis, MN 55455, USA

D. A. Chambers, MD
Department of Anesthesiology, St Joseph's Hospital, Atlanta,
Georgia, USA

M. F. Charnock, FRCS, MRCOG
Department of Obstetrics and Gynaecology, John Radcliffe
Hospital, Oxford OX3 9DU, England, UK

B. A. Clark, BS
Department of Obstetrics and Gynecology, University of
Minnesota Medical School, 420 Delaware Street SE,
Minneapolis, MN 55455, USA

L. A. Clayton, MD
Department of Obstetrics and Gynecology, Meharry Medical
College, Nashville, Tennessee, USA

W. T. Creasman, MD
Department of Gynecologic Oncology, Duke University Medical
School, Durham, North Carolina, USA

E. R. Davies, FRCPE, DMRD, FRCR
Department of Radiodiagnosis, University of Bristol, Bristol,
England, UK

R. L. Davies, MSc
Department of Radiology, Welsh National School of Medicine,
Heath Park, Cardiff, Wales, UK

G. Delgado, MD
Division of Gynecologic Oncology, Department of Obstetrics
and Gynecology, Georgetown University School of Medicine,
3800 Reservoir Road NW, Washington DC 20007, USA

I. D. Duncan, FRCOG
Department of Obstetrics and Gynaecology, Ninewells Hospital
and Medical School, Dundee, Scotland, UK

D. I. M. Farquharson, MRCOG, FRCSE
Department of Obstetrics and Gynaecology, University of
Edinburgh, Scotland, UK

S. Fletcher, BSc, MBChB, MIBiol, FRCPath
Department of Pathology, University of Edinburgh, Scotland, UK

E. W. Franklin, MD
Department of Gynecology, St Joseph's Hospital, Atlanta,
Georgia, USA

M. Fukushima, MD
Department of Obstetrics and Gynecology, University of
Minnesota Medical Center, 420 Delaware Street SE,
Minneapolis, MN 55455, USA

D. Gallup, MD
Department of Obstetrics and Gynecology, Naval Hospital,
Portsmouth, Virginia 23708, USA

W. E. Gibbons, MD
Reproductive Research Laboratory, St Luke's Episcopal Hospital
and Department of Obstetrics and Gynecology, Baylor College
of Medicine, Houston, Texas, USA

A. L. Goldson, MD
Department of Radiation Therapy, Howard University School of
Medicine, 2041 Georgia Avenue MW, Washington DC 20060,
USA

I. H. Gravelle, FRCR
Department of Radiology, Welsh National School of Medicine,
Heath Park, Cardiff, Wales, UK

T. W. Griffin, MD
Department of Medicine, University of Massachusetts Medical
Center, 55 Lake Avenue North, Worcester, MA 01605, USA

K. Griffiths, BSc, PhD
Tenovus Institute for Cancer Research, Welsh National School of
Medicine, Heath Park, Cardiff CF4 4XX, Wales, UK

N. F. Hacker, MD
Division of Gynecologic Oncology, UCLA School of Medicine,
Center for Ovarian Cancer, Johnsson Comprehensive Cancer
Care Center, Los Angeles, California 90024, USA

P. Heller, MD
Department of Obstetrics and Gynecology, Uniformed Services
University of Health Sciences, Bethesda, Maryland 20814, USA

W. J. Henderson, FRMS
Tenovus Institute for Cancer Research, Welsh National School of
Medicine, Heath Park, Cardiff, CF4 4XX, Wales, UK

H. Homesley, MD
Department of Gynecologic Oncology, Bowman Gray University,
Winston-Salem, North Carolina, USA

W. Hoskins, MD
Department of Obstetrics and Gynecology, Uniformed Services
University of Health Sciences, Bethesda, Maryland 20814, USA

R. E. Hunter, MD
Department of Obstetrics and Gynecology, University of
Massachusetts Medical Center, Worcester, MA 01605, USA

T. Iversen, MD, PhD
Department of Gynaecology, Norwegian Radium Hospital,
Montebello Oslo 3, Norway

C. A. Joslin, MB, BS, FRCR, DMRT
University Department of Radiotherapy, Cookridge Hospital,
Leeds LS16 6QB, England, UK

P. Kolstad, MD, PhD, FRCOG
Department of Gynaecology, Norwegian Radium Hospital,
Montebello, Oslo 3, Norway

C. G. Lacey, MD
Department of Obstetrics and Gynecology, University of San
Francisco, San Francisco, California, USA

L. D. Lagasse, MD
Division of Gynecologic Oncology, UCLA School of Medicine,
Center for Ovarian Cancer, Johnsson Comprehensive Cancer
Care Center, Los Angeles, California 90024, USA

T. Lai, MSc, MIBiol
Department of Surgery, University of Bristol, Bristol, England,
UK

M. Lawless, MSc
Department of Community Medicine and General Practice,
Gibson Laboratories Building, Radcliffe Infirmary, Oxford OX2
6HE, England, UK

P. M. Lenehan, FRCSI, MRCOG
National Maternity Hospital, Dublin, Ireland

R. S. Leuchter, MD
Division of Gynecologic Oncology, UCLA School of Medicine,
Los Angeles, California, USA

J. R. B. Livingstone, FRCOG, FRCSE
Department of Obstetrics and Gynaecology, University of
Edinburgh, Scotland, UK

W. H. McBride, PhD, MRCPath
Department of Radiation Oncology, UCLA Center for Health
Sciences, Los Angeles, California 90024, USA

N. Maitland, PhD
Department of Pathology, University of Bristol, England, UK

S. R. Mogelnicki, MD
Department of Anesthesiology, St Joseph's Hospital, Atlanta,
Georgia, USA

J. G. Moore, MD
Department of Obstetrics and Gynecology, UCLA School of
Medicine, Los Angeles, California, USA

D. Morris, MRCOG, MRACOG
Department of Obstetrics and Gynaecology, University of
Bristol, Bristol, England, UK

H. B. Morris, BSc, MBChB
Department of Pathology, University of Oxford, England, UK

C. P. Morrow, MD
Department of Gynecologic Oncology, University of Southern
California Medical School, Los Angeles, California, USA

D. Moyer, MD
Reproductive Research Laboratory, St Luke's Episcopal Hospital
and Department of Obstetrics and Gynecology, Baylor College
of Medicine, Houston, Texas, USA

K. Nieberg, MD
Department of Pathology, UCLA School of Medicine, Center for
Ovarian Cancer, Johnsson Comprehensive Cancer Care Center,
Los Angeles, California 90024, USA

T. Okagaki, MD, PhD
Department of Obstetrics and Gynecology, University of
Minnesota, Medical School, 420 Delaware Street SE,
Minneapolis, MN 55455, USA

R. Park, MD
Department of Obstetrics and Gynecology, Uniformed Services
University of Health Sciences, Bethesda, Maryland 20814, USA

E. S. Petrilli, MD
Division of Gynecologic Oncology, Department of Obstetrics
and Gynecology, Georgetown University School of Medicine,
3800 Reservoir Road NW, Washington DC 20007, USA

C. G. Pierrepoint, BVSc, PhD, FRCVS
Tenovus Institute for Cancer Research, Welsh National School of
Medicine, Heath Park, Cardiff CF4 4XX, Wales, UK

T. Poth, MPH
Division of Gynecologic Oncology, UCLA School of Medicine,
Center for Ovarian Cancer, Johnsson Comprehensive Cancer
Care Center, Los Angeles, California 90024, USA

R. A. Potish, MD
Department of Therapeutic Radiology, University of Minnesota
Hospitals, Minneapolis, MN 55455, USA

J. L. Powell, MD
Department of Gynecologic Oncology, Baystate Medical Center,
Springfield, Massachusetts, USA

J. M. Price, PhD
Department of Obstetrics and Gynecology, University of
Massachusetts, Medical Center, Worcester, MA 01605, USA

J. K. Pye, FRCS
Department of Surgery, Welsh National School of Medicine,
Heath Park, Cardiff, Wales, UK

S. D. Reich, MD
Department of Medicine and Pharmacology, University of
Massachusetts Medical Center, Worcester, MA 01605, USA

B. Resnick, AB
Division of Gynecologic Oncology, UCLA School of Medicine,
Center for Ovarian Cancer, Johnsson Comprehensive Cancer
Care Center, Los Angeles, California 90024, USA

G. E. Smart, FRCOG, FRCSE
Department of Obstetrics and Gynaecology, University of
Edinburgh, Edinburgh, Scotland, UK

G. S. Sykes, FRACOG, MRCOG
Department of Obstetrics and Gynaecology, University of
Oxford, England, UK

M. O. Symes, MD
Department of Surgery, University of Bristol, England, UK

G. M. Turner, FRCOG
Department of Obstetrics and Gynaecology, University of
Bristol, England, UK

L. B. Twiggs, MD
Department of Obstetrics and Gynecology, University of
Minnesota Medical School, 420 Delaware Street, SE,
Minneapolis, MN 55455, USA

M. P. Vessey, MD, FRCPE
Department of Community Medicine and General Practice,
Gibson Laboratories Building, Radcliffe Infirmary,
Oxford OX2 6HE, England, UK

E. Weiser, MD
Department of Obstetrics and Gynecology, Uniformed Services
University of Health Sciences, Bethesda, Maryland 20814, USA

E. Yordan, MD
Section of Gynecologic Oncology, Rush-Presbyterian, St. Luke's
Medical Center, Chicago, Illinois, USA

General

1 · Host Resistance to Cancer

W.H. McBride

Clinicians and research workers interested in cancer prefer to believe that tumours are influenced by a variety of host mechanisms, rather than being totally autonomous. Host resistance to cancer has long had particular appeal, because one day we might be able to control or even cure the disease by boosting or awakening host defences. Thus, in a report published in the 1806 edition of the *Edinburgh Medical and Surgical Journal* [1], 20 years before the discovery of the cell, a committee for the investigation of cancer asked: What factors dispose to cancer? What is the nature of precancerous changes? What is the significance of lymph node reactions?, and is there 'any native or acquired habit of the body that may dispose to or resist the influence of cancer?' In 1909 Ehrlich [2] suggested that 'if these (immune) mechanisms did not exist, we could expect that carcinomas would appear with enormous frequency.'

Burnet in 1957 [3] and Thomas 2 years later [4] crystallised the idea of host resistance to cancer in the process which Burnet called 'immunological sur-veillance'. Surveillance was by specific T cells which eliminated frequently arising neoplasms, and overt cancer was seen as a consequence of failure of the T cell system. In recent years this theory has been extensively reappraised and found wanting—not because it is necessarily completely wrong, but because it is too restrictive and is of little relevance to clinical cancer and its treatment.

Many mechanisms besides T cells are now known to be able to resist neoplastic growth and spread. The mechanism that is important will vary with the tumour, but three crucial questions must be asked: How effective is each mechanism? Under what circumstances does it operate? How can its efficiency be enhanced by therapeutic agents? Answers to these questions are required if immunotherapy is to gain a place as a treatment and if optimism in this line of research is to be justified. This article seeks to answer the questions. The examples used are highly selective, and the opinions expressed are personal.

Natural Immunity to Cancer

Awareness of the importance of natural immune mechanisms in cancer has been growing since the early 1970s, when leucocytes taken from normal individuals were found to lyse cancer cells in vitro. Similar mechanisms have been shown to operate in vivo.

Natural cytotoxicity is a property shared by subsets of macrophages, granulocytes and lymphocytes (NK or NC lymphocytes). Most, but not all, natural cytotoxic lymphocytes are large granular cells. They display considerable heterogeneity but in general appear to be distant relatives of classical T cells [5, 6,]. Little is known about the nature of cytotoxic granulocytes [7]. Cells of the mononuclear phagocyte system that display natural cytotoxicity are probably relatively immature [8].

Despite obvious differences between natural cytotoxic cells between and even within different lineages, it is probably worth emphasising the similarities between these cells, and asking to what extent they act and interact as a system to combat cancer in vivo.

Natural cytotoxic cells of all types show a distinct preference for binding neoplastic as opposed to normal cells. Unlike specific lymphocytes, they do not display specificity for the antigenic nature of the target. Instead the recognition system of lymphocytes [9,10], and possibly also that of macrophages [11], seems to involve lectin-like molecules that bind to tumour cell glycoconjugates [12]. This system could confer a pattern of broad specificity on the interactions, with each effector cell capable of binding perhaps several different targets. It should be stressed that it is not known how general this recognition system is. It may well differ depending upon which subset a cell belongs to and its differentiation and activation status.

Antibody may provide a more sophisticated, specific recognition system by which these cells can operate. All natural cytotoxic cells possess receptors that bind the Fc region of antigen-reacted immunoglobulin. With these receptors they can recognise antibody-coated target cells and trigger antibody-dependent cellular cytotoxicity (ADCC). In most respects, NK-NC cells seem to belong to the same lymphocyte subset as the 'K' cells and 'null cells' responsible for lymphocyte-mediated ADCC [13], and it is likely that the macrophage and granulocyte subsets involved in natural cytotoxicity can also mediate ADCC.

Following binding, neoplastic target cells are killed by a lytic extracellular mechanism, provided, of course, that the effector cells have a lytic apparatus to which the target cells are sensitive. Several possibly cytolytic mechanisms exist. The predominant one may vary with the subset of cells and their differentiation and activation status. The heterogeneity observed in natural cytotoxic cell populations could determine functional heterogeneity. Heterogeneity may be an advantage and provide broad activity against a wide range of targets.

Natural cytotoxicity is under both positive and negative regulation. Signals that boost activity generally fall into two major classes. One class is produced by lymphocytes in response to antigenic or mitogenic challenge. Several such 'lymphokine' factors are active. The other classes are produced as a result of direct interaction of materials like lipopolysaccharide and concanavalin A with the effector cells. Potentially important mediators of cytotoxicity are the interferons, some of which are lymphokines while others can be produced by a variety of cells

[14]. It is possible that several of the factors affecting cytotoxicity actually operate by first stimulating interferon synthesis, interferon being one of the final mediators in a pathway of responses [15]. Although interferon can act on more than one cell type, e.g. NK cells, macrophages and cytotoxic T cells [16], other mediators may be more cell-specific in their effects [17].

The phenotype and functions of natural cytotoxic cells are frequently altered following boosting or activation. For example, the range of targets NK cells can kill may change [13]. Macrophages may also change their phenotype and function following activation, activated macrophages being cytotoxic for tumour cells in a very non-specific fashion [18]. These phenotypic and functional alterations are probably the result of cell differentiation or the activation of existing cells.

Natural cytotoxicity is also under negative regulatory control. It can be depressed by factors such as PGE_2. The production of negative regulatory signals by some tumours may allow them to escape the attentions of host cytotoxic cells in vivo.

The crucial question of how important natural immunity is to the growth and spread of cancer in vivo has yet to be fully answered. However, Heberman and co-workers have shown that mouse strains differ in their levels of NK cell reactivity in vitro [19]. Mouse strains with high NK activity generally show greater resistance than strains with low activity. In mice with low NK cell activity, the metastatic capability of tumours is enhanced. Agents that boost the natural cytotoxic mechanism enhance resistance to the growth of injected tumour cells.

It can be concluded from these preliminary results that, in the absence of a specific immune response, natural cytotoxic cells constitute a primitive mechanism for dealing with a limited number of tumour cells. They may therefore prevent establishment of metastases, but there is no evidence that they can eradicate tumour foci once they are established.

Since tumours are transplantable, the system can readily be swamped by excess tumour cells. Furthermore, because the number of cells that have to be injected in order to generate a tumour differs enormously, it seems likely that the efficiency of the system is highly dependent upon the nature of the tumour. The potential of immunotherapy using agents which boost natural cytotoxic mechanisms is thus limited.

Before leaving the topic, it is worth speculating why we possess natural cytotoxicity. Most neoplasms arise in the post-reproductive years and thus exert little selective pressure. It is unlikely, therefore, that cytotoxic cells have developed primarily to combat cancer. They undoubtedly are effective against pathogens, and this may be their raison d'être. However, NK cells [20], and occasionally macrophages [21], have been found to kill fetal fibroblasts and certain haemotopoietic and lymphopoietic cells [22]. Thus natural cytotoxic cells may control the development of normal tissues. There are similarities between tumour cells and progenitor cells for normal tissues and it is not hard to imagine how they might share recognition structures, such as fetal antigens that could be recognised by natural cytotoxic cells.

Acquired Immunity to Cancer

Complementary to, and interacting with, natural immune mechanisms are those that are boosted specifically by antigen to give acquired immunity. However, it is still questionable whether human tumours have antigens recognisable as foreign by the host.

The development of monoclonal antibodies for the serological analysis of human tumour cell surfaces is the only way that unique serologically defined antigens are likely to be demonstrated on tumours. The source of such antibodies would, of course, be the B cells of the host, but the production of monoclonal antibodies suitable for demonstrating reactivity against tumour antigens is technically difficult: appropriate monoclonal antibody production demands, as its first step, the hybridisation of B cells with human plasmacytoma cells, and human plasmacytoma lines capable of this have only recently become available [23]. At present, monoclonal antibodies to human tumours are raised largely by hetero-immunisation and inevitably react mainly with species- or organ-specific antigens. Of those that do react preferentially with tumours, most, if not all, show no absolute tumour specificity and probably recognise developmental or differentiation antigens. Interestingly, they tend to demonstrate marked heterogeneity of antigen expression by cells within a tumour [24]. In general, while monoclonal antibodies will prove invaluable for immunodiagnostics, radio-immunolocalisation and drug-antibody targetting, they are unlikely, with rare exceptions [25], to prove themselves as effective therapeutic agents. Passively transferred antibody does not often cause tumour regression and, paradoxically, more often stimulates tumour growth [26].

In animal models T cells are known to be more potent than antibody in causing tumour regression and it is therefore important to know whether patients make specific T cell-mediated responses to their tumours. The demonstration of tumour-specific antigens by serological means does not help us to answer this question. The reason is that T cells have a narcissistic obsession with self HLA molecules. They respond to antigen only when complexed to self HLA, which is not what antibody normally binds.

The interaction of foreign antigen with their self HLA molecules is essential for the generation of an immune response. Furthermore, the class of HLA molecule involved (I or II) determines the type of response. Loss or down-regulation of HLA determinants, which has been reported for some human tumours [27], could be a means by which tumours escape the attentions of T cells. Other escape routes might be the refusal of tumour-specific antigens to associate with the correct HLA components, or such antigens might mimic, or be, cell-interaction molecules which suppress or interfere with the immune system [28]. Because of the above considerations, functional T cell assays must be performed with care, using lymphocytes and tumour cells from the same patient. Such assays are tedious and difficult to perform. Furthermore, there is disagreement as to what type of cell-mediated responses can cause tumour regression [29].

There are two basic forms of cell-mediated immunity which involve different T cell subsets—cytotoxic T cells and delayed-type hypersensitivity T cells. The latter release lymphokines which recruit and activate macrophages to function as the final effector arm. Both these responses can probably cause tumour regression, although conclusive experiments, particularly on the role of cytotoxic T cells, have not yet been performed. These and other problems in identifying the nature of the cytotoxic cells have led to much criticism of the many reports which suggest that lymphocytes from cancer patients respond to their tumour in functional T cell assays [30]. However, two important recent advances have been made which have helped to clarify this issue. Monoclonal antibodies now allow the identification of human T cell subsets with different functions, and, using T cell growth factor (a lymphokine), it is possible to clone individual functional T cell units. The results from studies employing these techniques show that a reasonable percentage of patients have T cells that can respond specifically to their own tumour in vitro either with proliferation or with cytotoxicity [31]. In time these studies will be extended to analyse the antigens that are being recognised, provide evidence on the uniqueness or cross-reactivity of these antigens and identify the reasons why only some individuals appear capable of responding. Only when responses can be analysed at this level will immunotherapy to eliminate tumour deposits in individual cancer patients begin to show promise.

Conclusions

In the past decade, out of the theories of immunological surveillance, a realistic general approach to host resistance in cancer has been developed. Questions such as whether cancer is a common occurrence held in check by an immune system that has as its main aim in life the destruction of aberrant cells are avoided in favour of questions more relevant to the treatment of cancer patients. A mark of the new approach is recognition of the diversity of anti-tumour responses and heterogeneity within each response. Each patient is seen to have a unique and ever-changing blend of responses. Some of these are beneficial, some harmful and some without effect. The overall composition of the response is determined by many factors. The effector mechanisms are regulated by various host cell–cell interactions and by soluble mediators that dictate the differentiation and activation status of the cells and hence their functional expression. The balance will be affected by tumour cell antigens and products and also by clinical intervention with drugs, surgery and radiotherapy.

The heterogeneity of host resistance mechanisms makes the disappointing results of the immunotherapy trials performed in the 1970s scarcely surprising. Only with careful step-by-step investigation of the immune responses in individual cancer patients and choice of a therapeutic regime tailored to that patient's needs, can we hope to assess the potential contribution of immunotherapy to cancer treatment.

References

1. Shimkin MB (1967) Thirteen questions: Some historical outlines for cancer research. J Natl Cancer Inst 19:295–298
2. Himmelweit F (ed) (1957) The collected papers of Paul Ehrlich, vol 2. Pergamon Press, London p 559
3. Burnet FM (1957) Cancer—A Biological Approach III. Viruses associated with neoplastic conditions. Br Med J I:841–847
4. Thomas (1959) In: Cellular and humoral aspects of hyper-sensitivity. Hoeber-Harper, New York, p 529

5. Herberman RB (ed) (1980) Natural cell-mediated immunity against tumours. Academic Press, New York London
6. Brooks C (1983) Reversible induction of natural killer cell activity in cloned murine cytotoxic T lymphocytes. Nature 305:155–158
7. Korec S (1980) In Herberman RB (ed) Natural cell-mediated immunity against tumours. Academic Press, New York London
8. Mantovani A, Peri G, Polentarutti N, Allavena P, Bordignon C, Sessa C, Mangioni C (1980) In: Herberman RB (ed) Natural cell-mediated immunity against tumours. Academic Press, New York London
9. Henney CS (1981) Do natural killer cells function through recognition of glycoconjugates on target cell membranes? In: Saunders JP (ed) Fundamental mechanisms of human cancer. Elsevier-North Holland, New York, pp 465–476
10. Stutman CPC (1980) Natural cytotoxic cells against solid tumours in mice: Blocking of cytotoxicity by D-mannose. Proc Natl Acad Sci 77:2895–2898
11. Pointek GE, Gronberg A, Ahrlund-Richter L, Keissling R, Hengarthner H (1982) NK-patterned binding expressed by non-NK mouse leukocytes. Int J Cancer 30:225–229
12. Weir DM, Grahame LM, Ogmundsdottir HM (1979) Binding of mouse peritoneal macrophages to tumour cells by a 'lectin-like' macrophage receptor. J Clin Lab Immunol 2:51–54
13. Koren HS, Herberman RB (1983) Natural-killing—Past and future (summary of workshop on natural killer cells). J Natl Cancer Inst 70:785–786
14. Toy JL (1983) The interferons. Clin Exp Immunol 54:1–13
15. Kawase I, Brooks CG, Kuriboyashi K, Olabuenaga S, Newman W, Gillis S, Henry C (1983) Interleukin 2 induces interferon production: participation of macrophages and NK-like cells. J Immunol 131:228–292
16. Wong GHW, Clark-Lewis I, McKinn-Breschkin JL, Harris AW, Schrader JW (1983). Interferon induces enhanced expression of Ia and H-2 antigens on B lymphoid macrophage and myeloid cell lines. J Immunol 131:788–793
17. Gemsa D, Debatin K, Kramer W, Kubelka C, Deimann W, Kees V, Krammer PH (1983) Macrophage-activating factors from different T cell clones induce distinct macrophage functions. J Immunol 131:833–844
18. Dougherty G, McBride WH (to be published) Macrophage heterogeneity. Immunol Today
19. Herberman RB , Timonen T, Ortaldo JR, Bennard GD, Kedar E, Gorelik E (1981) Characteristics of NK cells and their possible roles in resistance against tumour growth. In: Saunders JP (ed) Fundamental mechanisms in human cancer immunology. Elsevier-North Holland, New York, pp 499–512
20. Timonen T, Saksela E (1978) Human natural cell-mediated cytotoxicity against fetal fibroblasts. Cell Immunol 40:69–78
21. Jones JT, McBride WH, Weir DM (1975) The in vitro killing of syngeneic cells by peritoneal cells from adjuvant-stimulated mice. Cell Immunol 18:375–383
22. Moller G (1983) Elimination of allogeneic lymphocytes by mice. Immunol Rev 73:5–34
23. Kozbor D, Roder JC (1983) The production of monoclonal antibodies from human lymphocytes. Immunol Today 4:72–79
24. Egan ML, Henson DE (1982) Monoclonal antibodies and breast cancer. J Natl Cancer Inst 68:338–340
25. Beverley PCL (1982) Antibodies and cancer therapy. Nature 298:358–359
26. Prehn RT (1976) Do tumours grow because of an immune response of the host? Transplantation Rev 28:34–42
27. Sanderson AR, Beverley PCC (1983) Interferon, B_2 microglobulin in the pathway to malignancy. Immunol Today 4:211–212
28. Flood PM, De Leo AB, Old LJ, Gershon RK (1983) Relation of cell surface antigens on methylcholanthrene-induced fibrosarcomas to immunoglobulin heavy chain complex variable region-linked T cell interaction molecules. Proc Natl Acad Sci 80:1683–1687
29. Bahn A, Perry LL, Cantor H, McCluskey RT, Benacerraf B, Greane MI (1981) The role of T cell sets in the rejection of a methylcholanthrene-induced sarcoma (S1509a) in syngeneic mice. Am J Pathol 102:20–27
30. McBride WH (1981) Notes on the use of in vitro techniques for the assessment of cellular reactivity against tumours. In: Weir DM (ed) Handbook of immunology. Blackwells, Edinburgh Oxford, pp 1–14
31. Vose BM (1982) Quantitation of proliferative and cytotoxic precursor cells directed against human tumours: Limiting dilution analysis in peripheral blood and at the tumour site. Int J Cancer 30:135–142

2 · The Subrenal Capsule Assay as a Predictor of Tumour Response in Gynaecological Oncology

R.E. Hunter, T.W. Griffin, S.D. Reich, J.M. Price and A.E. Bogden

Introduction

Present cancer treatment requires selection of therapy for individual patients on the basis of clinical trials in large, heterogeneous populations of patients. Recent attention, however, has focused on the possibility of determining the susceptibility of an individual human malignancy to a therapeutic manoeuvre by means of prior laboratory testing of the tumour. The oestrogen receptor protein assay has demonstrated the clinical utility of this approach, by allowing selection of those patients more likely to respond to hormonal manipulation and exclusion of those patients unlikely to respond [1]. With regard to chemotherapeutic agents, attention has focused on the human tumour stem cell assay developed by Salmon and co-workers [2] and on the subrenal capsule assay developed by Bogden et al. [3].

The subrenal capsule (SRC) assay is an in vivo method which permits precise in situ measurements of human tumour fragments implanted under the renal capsule of mice. Studies using transplantation-established human tumour xenograft systems implanted in both athymic nude and in normal, immunocompetent mice have demonstrated that the SRC assay method is sensitive and precise enough to quantitate changes in xenograft size as early as 3 days after implantation [4]. These results suggest that the sensitivity and precision of the method would permit evasion of immunological complications in the normal mouse simply by limiting the assay to a 6-day period. The feasibility of utilising the normal mouse as a xenograft host for testing drugs against transplantation-established human tumours has been demonstrated [4]. Subsequently, it was shown that the 6-day

SRC assay could also be used for testing drugs against first transplant generation human tumours (surgical explants) in the normal, immunocompetent host [5].

To determine the morphological validity of the SRC assay, morphological examination of human cervical and endometrial carcinomas by light and electron microscopy has been performed, the findings indicating that the increase in tumour size observed at the end of the 6 days of the assay is due to an increase in tumour cell number. Such studies of the tumour fragments indicate the morphological changes to be consistent with viable tumour tissue. The transplanted tumours retain the histological characteristics of the original tumour.

In an attempt to determine the predictive accuracy of the assay in individual patient trials, we have performed 6-day SRC assays on more than 1500 consecutive tumour specimens at the University of Massachusetts Medical Centre and affiliated hospitals [8]. Hunter et al. reported a preliminary study on the responsiveness of gynaecological cancer to chemotherapeutic agents in the SRC assay and this report provides additional experience [9].

Methods and Materials

The basic SRC assay methodology has been described in previous publications [3].

Results

Table 2.1 presents the results of SRC assay of 1000 solid tumours of varying histopathological types. Eight hundred and fifty-eight, or 86%, of the assays could be evaluated as defined by a mean control, $\Delta TS \geqslant -0.5$ omu (ocular micrometer units). Reasons for selection of this criterion have been previously presented [5]. Rates of success in evaluation varied from 95% in breast cancer, to 63% in sarcoma. The number of assays obtained with gynaecological tumours in the SRC assay that can be evaluated is high, ranging from 91% for cervical carcinomas to 95% for endometrial carcinomas (Table 2.2).

The response rates of various neoplasms of the human female to clinically active chemotherapeutic agents have been obtained for 115 ovarian, 81 endometrial and 63 cervical carcinomas (Table 2.3), using the data only on assays that could be evaluated. A tumour was considered to be sensitive to a drug if the average regression was $\geqslant 25\%$. Responses varied from 9% to cisplatin in cervical carcinomas, to 60% to vincristine in ovarian carcinomas. At present it is not clear whether these rates reflect clinical response rates when optimal doses and schedules are used for each of these single agents in previously untreated patients with minimum tumour burdens.

Table 2.1. Evaluable assays by tumour type: 6-day SRC assay

Type of tumour (source of sample)[a]	Number of tumours tested in SRC assays	
	No. evaluable/ total tested	% evaluable
Breast	195/206	95
Lymphoma	83/98	85
Lung: Non-small cell	55/69	80
Small cell	9/12	75
Not reported	10/14	71
Ovarian	77/82	94
Endometrium	67/79	85
Colorectal	58/69	84
Cervix	52/58	90
Melanoma	26/35	74
Kidney	26/32	81
Sarcoma	17/27	63
Gastric	14/17	82
Unknown primary	44/53	83
Miscellaneous tumours ($<$ 10 assays/type) and non-malignant tissue	125/149	84
Total evaluable assays	858/1000	86

[a] All samples of solid tumour, either biopsy or surgical specimens. Evaluable assay = mean control growth $\geq$ −0.5 omu.

Table 2.2. Evaluable assay rate for gynaecological tumours in the SRC assay

Tumour type	Evaluable assay rate[a]	
	Evaluable/total	Percent
Ovarian	115/122	94
Endometrial	81/85	95
Cervical	63/69	91
Overall	259/276	94

[a] Evaluable assay = mean control $\geq$ −0.5 omu.

Table 2.3. Comparison of the response[a] of gynaecological tumours to clinically active chemotherapeutic agents (6-day SRC assay)

Chemotherapeutic agent	Tumour type		
	Ovarian (%)	Endometrial (%)	Cervical (%)
Vincristine	60	38	32
5-Fluorouracil	43	59	48
L-Phenylalanine mustard	36	43	
Cytoxan	38	39	33
Adriamycin	33	18	22
Methotrexate	45	32	31
Cisplatin	21	10	9

[a] A positive response = tumour regression $\geq$25%.

Retrospective Study

A retrospective analysis was made of 55 patients with malignancies who were treated with one or more chemotherapeutic agent which had been screened previously in an evaluable SRC assay against biopsy or surgical specimens of their tumours. Simultaneously, objective measurements of their disease response were made. These patients typically were previously untreated with chemotherapy and had relatively chemotherapeutic-sensitive tumours: breast (12), ovary (8), lymphoma (16), small cell lung cancer (3), myeloma (2), carcinoma of unknown primary (2), miscellaneous others (12). They were treated in a conventional manner with standard chemotherapeutic regimens. Assay results did not influence their treatment. Standard criteria of clinical tumour response and regression [7] were employed in assessment of treatment outcome. Activity in the assay was defined as a measurable regression of the tumour fragments ($\geqslant-0.5$ omu).

Fifty-five patients have provided 62 clinical trials for retrospective analysis. Histological types of these patients' tumours are presented in Table 2.4. Results of the analysis are presented in Table 2.5.

Of the 38 patients responding clinically to a drug combination, 37 were treated with drug combinations containing at least one drug indicated to be active in the assay. Of the 24 patients judged to be resistant clinically, 16 were treated with drug combinations containing no active agents in the assay. Of these 62 assay-clinical correlations, therefore, 37 were true-positives, 8 false-positives, 16 true-negatives and 1 false-negative.

This yields a sensitivity of clinical response of 0.97 for the assay, with a specificity of 0.33. Thus, the assay correctly identifies 97% of clinical responders and 67% of clinical non-responders (Table 2.6). The correlation between assay results and clinical outcome, calculated in this manner, is statistically significant ($P<0.0001$, Fisher Exact Test). Also by this method of analysis, the assay was predictive of clinical response in 37 of 45 trials (82%) and predictive of clinical resistance in 16 of 17 trials (94%), yielding an overall predictive accuracy of 85%.

Table 2.7 indicates the results of a retrospective study of ovarian cancer. The predictive accuracy of the assay in this study was 74%.

Table 2.4. Retrospective analysis: histological diagnoses

Lymphoma	16
Breast	12
Ovary	8
Lung (small cell)	3
Myeloma	2
Unknown primary	2
Others	12
	55

Table 2.5. Retrospective analysis: predictive accuracy of SRC assay

No. of patients	No. of correlations[a]	S/S	S/R	R/R	R/S
55	62	37	8	16	1

Predictive of clinical sensitivity	37/45 (82%)
Predictive of clinical resistance	16/17 (94%)
Overall predictive accuracy	53/62 (85%)

[a] Assay results/clinical results: $P < 0.0001$ (Fisher Exact Test)
S = drug sensitive
R = drug resistant

Table 2.6. Retrospective analysis: SRC assay/clinical response correlations

No. of patients	No. of clinical trials	Assay/clinical correlations[a]			
		S/S	R/S	R/R	S/R
55	62	37	1	16	8

Clinical responders:	True-positive (S/S)	37
	False-positive (R/S)	1
	Correctly identified	37/38 (97%)
Clinical non-responders:	True-negative (R/R)	16
	False-negative (S/R)	8
	Correctly identified	16/24 (67%)

[a] $P < 0.0001$ (Fisher Exact Test)

Table 2.7. Results of a retrospective study of the predictive accuracy of SRC assay in ovarian cancer.

No. of patients	Inevaluable assay		Too early	
34	3		4	
27	S/S	S/R	R/R	R/S
	16	3	4	4

Prospective Study

On the basis of the promising results of the retrospective analysis of the clinical correlations, a prospective study was initiated. All patients involved in this study had advanced metastatic disease. They were treated in a prospective fashion with the agent producing the greatest amount of growth inhibition or regression in the SRC assay. Chemotherapy was administered according to standard dosages and schedules. Eligibility requirements for protocol entry were: metastatic malignancy for which there is no standard therapy of clinical value, or which has become refractory to conventional therapy; an evaluable SRC assay; reproducible, objective measurement of disease; performance status of 3 or better; expected duration of survival of at least 8 weeks; and signed informed consent to an experimental study. Patients showing stable disease or partial response after two cycles of therapy were continued on single agent chemotherapy or switched to combination chemotherapy including the original agent and a second active

Table 2.8. SRC assay: histological types in prospective study

Unknown primary	7
Lymphoma	7
Lung carcinoma, small cell	3
non-small cell	6
Ovarian carcinoma	4
Cervical carcinoma	4
Sarcoma	4
Melanoma	4
Colon carcinoma	4
Endometrial carcinoma	1
Oesophageal carcinoma	1
Mesothelioma	1
Carcinoid	1
	47

agent, at the discretion of their attending physician. Patients showing progressive disease after one complete cycle of therapy were considered treatment failures and were withdrawn from the protocol. Standard definitions of response evaluation were employed [6].

Forty-seven patients with cancers refractory to chemotherapy have been entered in the prospective study. The histological types of these patients' tumours are present in Table 2.8. These 47 patients have provided 50 clinical trials. Six clinical trials (12%) were judged inevaluable for response: three patients suffered early death, one was lost to follow-up, one was entered with no measurable disease and one withdrew early because of drug toxicity. Also, four clinical trials are too early for evaluation (owing to recent patient entry). All responses required the standard criteria for partial response, complete response and progressive disease.

Fourteen of 37 patients (38%) and 17 of 40 clinical courses (42%) showed partial or complete response. The median duration of response in all patients was 4 months. The probability of patient response showed a strong relationship to the percentage of fragment regression in the assay. For the small group of patients with 60% tumour fragment regression by day 6 (≥ 3.0 omu change in tumour size), seven of eight patients responded. Moreover, duration of tumour response seemed clearly related to single agent drug activity in the assay. Responses were shortlived in the group with ≥ 3.0 omu of single agent activity (median duration of remission, 6 weeks), in contrast to responses in patients with a greater degree of regression (median duration of remission, 8 months) (Table 2.9). Patients in the latter group also demonstrated significantly increased survival as compared with non-responders to chemotherapy.

Table 2.9. Clinical response rates and duration of response in relation to tumour regression in assay (prospective, decision-aiding trials)

Tumour regression in SCR assay	Clinical response rate[a]		Median duration of response
≥ 3.0 omu	6/7	86%	8 months
≤ 2.9 omu	8/30	27%	6 weeks
All regressions	14/30	38%	4 months

[a]   7/37 (19%) patients highly responsive in assay.

Conclusion

In summary, the SRC assay is an in vivo test in mice which can rank the effectiveness of chemotherapeutic agents against individual human tumours. It is a reliable assay and can be completed within a clinically useful time frame. The assay reflects the heterogeneity of tumours within specific tumour histological types. The SRC assay is currently undergoing clinical study as a potential clinical test to predict which drug or drugs will be most effective against a tumour in an individual patient.

References

1. McGuire WL, Horowitz KB, Zava DT et al. (1978) Hormones in breast cancer: Update 1978. Metabolism 27:487–501
2. Hamburger AW, Salmon SE (1977) Primary bioassay of human tumor stem cells. Science 197: 461–463
3. Bogden AE, Cobb WR, Kelton DE, LePage DJ, Remington K, Cote TH (1978) A six-day subrenal capsule assay for drug screening using the normal immunocompetent mouse as host for human tumor xenografts (Abstr). Proc AACR and ASCO 19:105
4. Bogden AE, Haskell PM, LePage DJ, Kelton DE, Cobb WR, Esber HJ (1979) Human tumor xenografts implanted under the renal capsule of normal immunocompetent mice. Exp Cell Biol 47:281–293
5. Bogden AE, Cobb WR, LePage DJ et al. (1981) Chemotherapy responsiveness of human tumors as first transplant generation xenografts in the normal mouse: 6-day subrenal capsule assay. Cancer 48: 10–20
6. Bogden AE, Cobb WR, LePage DL, Kelton DE (1981) Reproducibility of chemotherapy response profiles of human tumor explants in the 6-day subrenal capsule (SRC) assay (Abstr). Proc AACR and ASCO 22:224
7. Miller AB, Hoogstratten B, Staguet M, Winkler A (1981) Reporting results of cancer treatment. Cancer 47:207–214
8. Griffin TW, Bogden AE, Reich SD et al. (to be published) Initial clinical trials of the subrenal capsule assay as a predictor of tumor response to chemotherapy. Cancer
9. Hunter RE, Reich SD, Griffin TW, Bogden AE (1982) Responsiveness of gynecologic tumors to chemotherapeutic agents in the six-day subrenal capsule assay. Gynecol Oncol 14:298–306

Cervix

3 · The Viral Aetiology of Cancer of the Cervix

N. Maitland

Introduction

To establish the viral aetiology of a particular tumour there are several criteria which must be fulfilled (Table 3.1). Firstly, it must be shown that the disease is rigorously associated with infection by the virus in question. This type of sero-epidemiology is open to misinterpretation on several counts; viz. the viral infection may be a consequence, rather than the cause of the tumour, because of the altered immunological status of the patient. Equally the viral infection may simply be a passenger, in combination with another type of infection, which itself may be the actual cause of the tumour.

Secondly, detection of viral genetic information and gene products in the actual tumours by nucleic acid hybridisation and immunofluorescence or immunoperoxidase techniques has a significant advantage over the sero-epidemiological approach. However, the order of acquisition of the viral genes, i.e. before or after the initial transformation event, is still difficult to determine. One possible approach, particularly with a disease like carcinoma of the cervix which may be divided into a series of well defined stages, would be to assay for the presence of the viral information during tumour development.

Thirdly, the virus in question must be shown to have oncogenic potential both in vitro (Table 3.2) and in vivo, the latter necessarily in laboratory animals. Once

Table 3.1. Determination of viral aetiology

1. Is the viral infection epidemiologically linked to the incidence of the tumour?
2. Can viral gene products be detected in patients with the tumour?
3. Does the virus have in vitro oncogenic potential?
4. Does vaccination against the primary viral infection reduce the incidence of the tumour?

Table 3.2. Parameters of in vitro cell transformation by tumour viruses

---

1. Does treatment of primary tissue culture cells with virus result in cells with altered growth characteristics (morphological transformation)?
2. Do the transformed cells retain specific viral genes?
3. Can fragments of the viral chromosome also produce morphological transformation when introduced into primary cells?
4. Are the retained viral genes expressed normally in the transformed cells (messenger RNA, antigens)?
5. Will the morphologically transformed cells produce tumours in syngeneic or immunodeficient animals?

---

again such studies are open to criticism since they are mostly performed in heterologous systems, e.g. human viruses in rodent cells. A true animal model of tumorigenesis should therefore employ a homologous system such as human virus in primary human cells. The other defect in most in vitro transformations is their reliance on either established tissue culture cell lines or fibroblastic cell cultures as the targets for transformation when the tumour under study is a carcinoma of epithelial cell origin. It must be said in defence of the latter approach that, by using cells which are already partially transformed (e.g. NIH3T3 mouse cells), these experiments overcome the requirement for at least two individual mutagenic events to produce a tumorigenic cell phenotype.

Lastly, and possibly most importantly, would be prognostic studies concerned with prevention of the viral infection in the general population. The growing efficacy of antiviral vaccines should permit such studies which, if reduction in the incidence of the tumour followed elimination of the primary viral infection, would present the best possible evidence for an aetiological relationship. Again, misinterpretation is possible, however, since vaccination is often accompanied by a change in general health education which may eliminate other unknown aetiological factors.

With these guidelines, it is now proposed to review the evidence for and against a number of human viruses (listed in Table 3.3) as oncogenic agents in human epithelial neoplasia, with special reference to carcinoma of the cervix.

Specific Viral Oncogenic Agents

Herpes Simplex Virus

Considerable epidemiological evidence has been published linking, as an aetiological agent, herpes simplex virus (HSV), and particularly HSV2, to human squamous carcinoma of the cervix. The evidence in favour of this virus as an aetiological agent has been extensively reviewed by Rapp [1]. However, some of the more recent sero-epidemiological studies by Mendis and co-workers, who employed defined antisera, have resulted in rather open-ended conclusions [2], and Wenczer et al. have published data which implicate HSV in adenocarcinoma of the cervix [3]. The earliest sero-epidemiological studies also indicated that HSV2 was the genital variant, whereas the oral variant was HSV1. The site of

Table 3.3. Human viruses associated with cervical intra-epithelial neoplasia

1. Herpes simplex viruses types 1 and 2
2. Human cytomegalovirus
3. Human papillomaviruses (types 6, 11, 16 and 18)
(4. Retroviruses)

isolation was therefore a major factor in the design of the subsequent experiments, which often used the relative titres of serum antibodies against HSV1/HSV2 to establish the significance of these results with respect to incidence of carcinoma of the cervix. However, there is now a growing amount of evidence, obtained by comparison of the different DNA restriction endonuclease fingerprints of HSV1 and 2, that HSV1 is isolated from a large proportion of genital lesions [4]. This suggests, if the sero-epidemiological results are correct, that there is a hitherto undiscovered fundamental difference between the transformation specificities of HSV types 1 and 2. The different map locations of the transforming regions of HSV1 and 2 may provide a clue to this difference, otherwise HSV1 is as likely as HSV2 to be the aetiological agent in carcinoma of the cervix.

More conclusive evidence for viral involvement has been provided by the detection of viral antigens [5] and viral nucleic acid [6,7,8,9] in frozen sections of dysplastic and tumour tissue. Using monospecific antisera a number of non-structural viral polypeptides have been identified in the carcinoma tissue. By hybridisation a number of workers have identified transcription of RNA from specific regions of the HSV2 genome in a proportion of the dysplastic and carcinomatous tissues [6,7,8,9]. Workers have demonstrated the presence of a small fragment of HSV2 DNA in a small number of adenocarcinomas of the cervix, but no such DNA was detected in a larger number of squamous cell carcinomas [10, and J. K. McDougall 1983, personal communication]. These results were in direct contrast to the results of in situ hybridisations to frozen sections of cervical tissue using HSV2 DNA probes, where adenocarcinomas were uniformly negative while a high percentage of the squamous cell carcinomas appeared to contain HSV2-specific RNA [9]. Recent research in our own laboratory has suggested that the RNA detected by in situ hybridisation was, in fact, cell-specific RNA which was transcribed to excess in the more rapidly dividing tumour cells. This RNA contains nucleotide base sequences which are homologous to HSV DNA [6,11], and was not present in sufficient quantities in the normal tissues to be detected in the hybridisation reactions. As increasingly sensitive probes for both viral RNA and antigens (cloned subfragments of the viral genome and monoclonal antibodies respectively) are made available, the possibility of cross-reaction with cellular homologues will increase, and future experiments of this type must be carefully controlled (e.g. by using biopsies of normal and tumour tissue from the same patient in all experiments).

Since the first demonstration of the ability of HSV to cause oncogenic transformation of tissue culture cells [12], a considerable amount of effort has been expended in attempts to locate the HSV genes and antigens responsible for cellular transformation. Many candidates have been proposed by several different laboratories [1,2,5,8,13,14] but even the briefest examination of the results will indicate the lack of cohesion in the final analysis. No single tumour antigen has been convincingly demonstrated and when transformations have been conducted with cloned individual viral DNA fragments, no single transforming sequence has been isolated, in contrast to the adenovirus and papovavirus systems [15]. In fact, no fewer than three non-contiguous sequences on the normally colinear genetic maps of HSV1 and HSV2 have been responsible for cellular transformation [13,16,17]. These results, and the recent work by D.A. Galloway et al. (1983, personal communication) which has elegantly demonstrated that fewer than 227 bases (and possibly 100 bases) of genetic information with incomplete protein coding potential are sufficient to initiate the transformation of tissue culture cells by HSV2, have led these and other investigators to reject the traditional 'transforming gene' hypothesis, in which expression of the viral gene to produce a functional protein is essential. Rather they have embraced the 'hit and run' hypothesis, proposed for HSV2 and cervical cancer by Skinner [14,18]. The latter mechanism suggests a viral mutagenic action, similar to that of chemical carcinogens, for which there is in fact some evidence [19, and B. Matz 1983, personal communication]. From the results of the in vitro transformation studies, it appears that HSV does have oncogenic potential but is unlikely to code for a T antigen type protein. Rather the insertion, temporary or otherwise, of a small piece of viral nucleic acid into the cellular chromosome is sufficient to cause the oncogenic change. It is the insertion and position of the viral gene, rather than its expression as protein, which are thought to be the factors responsible for the change in cellular phenotype. Whether this in vitro mechanism is applicable in vivo will be more difficult to decide, and only greater knowledge of the primary effects of mutagens (both chemical and viral) on cellular control processes at the genetic level will resolve this question. Were anti-HSV vaccination to effect a decrease in the incidence of cervical carcinoma, then a causative relationship would be more likely.

Cytomegalovirus

Cytomegalovirus, another human herpes virus, has been implicated as an aetiological agent in carcinoma of the cervix by studies similar to those described for HSV. Sero-epidemiological results indicated that patients with carcinoma generally had higher titres of antibodies against CMV than matched controls [20,21]. The presence of CMV genetic information in another human tumour (Kaposi's sarcoma) has been demonstrated [22 and D. Spector 1983, personal communication]. However, since a large proportion of the human population carries a latent CMV infection, it is probably not surprising that, under the immunodeficient conditions normally associated with Kaposi's sarcoma (such as the acquired immune deficiency syndrome, AIDS), reactivation of CMV takes place. The most recent results suggest that the CMV is probably present as a reactivated infection rather than as an oncogene [D. Spector 1983, personal communication].

In vitro studies have indicated that CMV has oncogenic potential in rodent cell systems [23], and studies employing purified viral DNA, transfected into rodent cells, have defined a small region of the genome which appears to be essential for in vitro transformation [24 and J.A. Nelson, 1983, personal communication]. Like the corresponding fragment of HSV, the CMV transforming region does not contain either 'start' signals for protein coding, or even a 'large open reading frame' in its genetic code, which means that it is not capable of producing an active protein. Thus again, like HSV, the possibility of a purely viral tumour antigen is unlikely, and viral mutagenesis is the more credible mechanism.

Since most of the human population carry antibodies against CMV, or even a latent virus infection, it is only under immunosuppressed conditions or in early childhood that the effects of viral infection are severe. Protection by immunisation would therefore mostly be confined to a boost of natural immunity, and could not in most cases be given sufficiently early to prevent the primary infection.

Human Papilloma Viruses

The benign human tumours caused by papilloma viruses have been known for many years and the oncogenic potential of a number of animal papilloma viruses has been well established. It was suggested by zur Hausen in 1976 [25] that benign tumours were capable of conversion to a malignant phenotype under appropriate stimuli. This hypothesis has been supported by the elegant demonstrations in epidermodysplasia verruciformis [26], juvenile multifocal laryngeal papillomas [27], and bovine alimentary tract carcinoma [28], that the action of a secondary mutagen on the benign papilloma cells can indeed convert them to a malignant phenotype. Papilloma virus infection is now found with increasing frequency in the human cervix. The koilocytic cells which are associated with many intra-epithelial lesions are readily identified by histological stains [29], and papilloma virus particles have been observed in such lesions by electron microscopy [30]. There is no direct evidence that these particular lesions convert with high frequency to a malignant phenotype, although the dysplasia is very similar to that preceding carcinoma in situ, and preliminary sero-epidemiological evidence has been published linking invasive squamous cell carcinoma of the cervix to the presence of antibody against HPV [31]. In recent years, with the increasing availability of HPV DNA probes, the search for HPV genomes in the cancer cells has been more successful [32,33]. The major difficulty in studies with the HPV has been the large number of serotypes of HPV and their relative uniqueness, which has meant that the use of, for example, an HPV1 probe to detect HPV6 sequences, is almost impossible except at low hybridisation stringencies. A number of HPV types have specifically been associated with human genital cancer, by detection of viral DNA in the tumour cells, viz. HPV 6, 11, 16 and 18 (see Table 3.4) and the number may be set to rise with the isolation of new HPV types. Of these, HPV16 is the most common type isolated from the human cervical carcinoma (zur Hausen 1983, personal communication), and the specific cloned DNA probes for this virus should allow a greater number of malignant tumours to be screened for the presence of the viral DNA. One interesting speculation is possible: if, as seems likely, one particular type of HPV is found in most carcinoma tissue (HPV16), whilst present in only a small minority of the premalignant lesions, then it may be possible to predict those patients at greater risk of developing carcinoma by determining the HPV serotype which they carry. The state of the HPV genome in the tumour cells is particularly interesting. Unlike most of the other DNA tumour viruses, and like Epstein-Barr virus, the HPV is found as an episomal double-stranded supercoiled circle of DNA, present in several copies per cell. Thus, the viral DNA has not become integrated into the host cell chromosomes [33].

Table 3.4. Detection of human papillomavirus DNA in human tissue extracts[a]

Human papilloma virus (serotype number)	% Detection in tissue of patients with			
	1 E.V.	2 Cond.	3 Dys.	4 Ca. Cervix
5	80	–	–	–
6	–	60	10	2
10	–	–	10	2
11	–	30	50	–
16	–	–	10	50
18	–	–	–	20

1   Epidermodysplasia verruciformis
2   Condylomata accuminata
3   Cervical dysplasia
4   Carcinoma of the cervix
[a]   Personal communication from H. zur Hausen (July 1983)

Burnett and Gallimore [34] have reported in vitro transformation of human keratinocytes with HPV1 DNA with continued presence and expression of the HPV genes. However, the identification of a single HPV transforming sequence of gene has not yet been reported.

Vaccination against HPV would be extremely difficult since the virus is able to persist in an unknown latent form for long periods, with subsequent reactivation under immunodeficient conditions. Only with more knowledge about the specific neutralisation of the many individual types of HPV would a vaccination strategy be possible and only by prevention of the primary infection could it possibly be successful.

Retroviruses

This topic has been dealt with in detail in the literature and the reader is referred to a recent review in Nature by Duesberg [35]. Whether the retrovirus oncogenes are truly viral genes is doubtful, but the retroviruses are certainly capable of inserting oncogenes at active chromosomal locations in human cells, e.g. in Burkitt's lymphoma and promyelocytic leukaemia [36,37]. Identification of similar chromosomal rearrangements and activation of a particular oncogene which is characteristic for carcinoma of the cervix have not yet been reported, although a recent review by Yunis [38] has indicated that there may be a carcinoma-specific chromosomal break on human chromosome No 1. This break does not, however, appear to coincide with the location of the 'ras oncogene', which has been shown to be active in other human carcinomas [39].

Conclusions

While considerable time, money and effort have been expended in the determination of a viral aetiology for carcinoma of the cervix, the nature of the interactions of the candidate viruses and the tumour is by no means certain. A two-stage carcinogenesis model [40], which takes into account the involvement of both HPV and HSV, has recently been proposed. It has also been shown that HSV [41] is capable of reactivating latent retroviral genes, and studies reported very recently [42] indicate that such a two-stage model with independent roles for different oncogenes and DNA tumour viruses can be demonstrated in vitro. Therefore future studies should perhaps concentrate on the interactions between a number of candidate initiators and promoters of oncogenesis in cervical tissue. In the longer term, the most beneficial approach would be to prevent or eliminate the primary viral infections, which are also unpleasant, and await any resultant decrease in the incidence of the tumour.

References

1. Rapp F (1982) The viral aetiology of cervical cancer. In: Oncology overview, International Cancer Research Data Bank program. National Cancer Institute, USA
2. Mendis LS, Best JM, Sonerath LI, Chiphangwi J, Vestergaard BF, Banatvala JE (1981) A geographical study of antibodies to membrane antigens of HSV2-infected cells and HSV2-specific antibodies in patients with cervical cancer. Int J Cancer 28:525–542
3. Wenczer J, Yaron-Schiffer O, Leventon-Kriss S, Modan M, Modan B (1981) Herpesvirus type 2 in adenocarcinoma of the uterine cervix: a possible association. Cancer 48:1497–1499
4. Smith IW, Maitland NJ, Peutherer JF, Robertson DHH (1981) Restriction enzyme analysis of herpesvirus type 2 DNA. Lancet II 1424
5. Dreesman GR, Burek J, Adam E, Kaufman RH, Melnick JL (1980) Expression of herpesvirus induced antigens in human cervical cancer. Nature 283:591–593
6. Maitland NJ, Kinross JH, Busuttil A, Ludgate SM, Smart GE, Jones KW (1981) The detection of DNA tumour virus specific RNA sequences in abnormal human cervical biopsies by in situ hybridization. J Gen Virol 55:123–137
7. McDougall JK, Galloway DA, Fenoglio CM (1980) Cervical carcinoma: Detection of herpes simplex virus RNA in cells undergoing neoplastic change. Int J Cancer 25:1–8
8. McDougall JK, Crum CP, Fenoglio CM, Goldstein LC, Galloway DA (1982) Herpesvirus specific RNA and protein in carcinoma of the uterine cervix. Proc Natl Acad Sci USA 79:3853–3857
9. Eglin RP, Sharp F, MacLean AB, MacNab JCM, Clements JB, Wilkie NM (1981) Detection of RNA complementary to herpes simplex virus DNA in human cervical squamous cell neoplasms. Cancer Res 41:3597–3603
10. Park M, Kitchener HC, MacNab JCM (1983) Detection of herpes simplex virus type 2 restriction fragments in human cervical carcinoma tissue. EMBO J 2:1029–1034
11. Peden K, Mounts P, Hayward GS (1982) Homology between mammalian cell DNA sequences and human herpes virus genomes detected by a hybridization procedure with a high complexity probe. Cell 31:71–80
12. Duff R, Rapp F (1971) Properties of hamster embryo fibroblasts transformed in vitro after exposure to ultraviolet irradiated herpes simplex virus type 2. J Virol 8:469–477
13. Camacho A, Spear PG (1978) Transformation of hamster embryo fibroblasts by a specific fragment of the herpes simplex virus genome. Cell 15:993–1002
14. Galloway DA, McDougall JK (1983) The oncogenic potential of herpes simplex viruses: Evidence for a 'hit and run' mechanism. Nature 302:21–24
15. Sharp PA (1979) Molecular biology of viral oncogenes. Cold Spring Harbor Symp Quant Biol 44:1305–1322
16. Reyes GR, LaFemina R, Hayward SD, Hayward GS (1979) Cold Spring Harbor Symp Quant Biol 44:629–641
17. Jariwalla RJ, Aurelian L, Ts'o PO (1980) Tumorigenic transformation induced by a specific fragment of DNA from herpes simplex virus type 2. Proc Natl Acad Sci USA 77:2279–2282
18. Skinner GR (1976) Transformation of primary hamster embryo fibroblasts by type 2 herpes simplex virus: Evidence for a 'hit and run' hypothesis. Br J Exp Pathol 57:361–376

19. Schlehofer JR, zur Hausen H (1982) Induction of mutations within the host cell genome by partially inactivated herpes simplex virus type 1. Virology 122:471–475
20. Melnick JL, Lewis R, Wimberley I, Kaufman RH, Adam E (1975) Association of cytomegalovirus (CMV) infection with cervical cancer: Isolation of CMV from cell cultures derived from cervical biopsy. Intervirology 10:115–119
21. Alexander ER, Chiang WT, Wei PY (1976) Association of cervical cytomegalovirus infection and dysplasia. In: Third International Symposium on detection and prevention of cancer, April 1976, New York
22. Giraldo G, Beth E, Huang ES (1980) Kaposi's sarcoma and its relationship to cytomegalovirus (CMV) III: CMV DNA and MV early antigens in Kaposi's sarcoma. Int J Cancer 26:23–29
23. Albrecht T, Rapp F (1973) Malignant transformation of hamster embryo fibroblasts following exposure to ultraviolet irradiated human cytomegalovirus. Virology 55:53–61
24. Nelson JA, Fleckenstein B, Galloway DA, McDougall JK (1982) Transformation of NIH3T3 cells with cloned fragments of human cytomegalovirus strain AD169. J Virol 43:83–91
25. zur Hausen H (1976) Condylomata acuminata and human genital cancer. Cancer Res 36:794
26. Orth G, Favre M, Breitberg F (1980) Epidermodysplasia verruciformis: A model for the role of papillomaviruses in human cancer. In: Essex M, Todaro G, zur Hausen H (eds) Viruses in naturally occurring cancer. Cold Spring Harbor Laboratory Press, NY, USA, pp 259–282
27. zur Hausen H (1977) Human papillomaviruses and their possible role in squamous cell carcinomas. Curr Top Microbiol Immunol 78:1–30
28. Jarrett WFH, McNeil PE, Laird HM, O'Neill BW, Murphy J, Campo MS, Moar MH (1980) Papillomaviruses in benign and malignant tumours of cattle. In: Essex M, Todaro G, zur Hausen H (eds) Viruses in naturally occurring cancer. Cold Spring Harbour Laboratory Press, NY, USA, pp 215–225
29. Fletcher S (1983) Histopathology of papilloma virus infection of the cervix uteri: The history, taxonomy, nomenclature and reporting of koilocytic dysplasias. J Clin Pathol 36:616–624
30. Meisels A, Roy M, Fortier M (1981) Human papilloma virus infection of the cervix: The atypical condyloma. Acta Cytol 25:7–16
31. Baird PJ (1983) Serological evidence for the association of papillomavirus and cervical neoplasia. Lancet II:17–18
32. Green M, Brackman KH, Sanders PR (1982) Isolation of human papilloma virus from a patient with epidermodysplasia verruciformis: Presence of related viral DNA genomes in human urogenital tumours. Proc Natl Acad Sci USA 79:4437–4441
33. Gissman L, Wolnik L, Ikenberg H, Koldovski U, Schnurch HG, zur Hausen H (1983) Human papilloma virus types 6 and 11 DNA sequences in genital and laryngeal papillomas and in some cervical cancers. Proc Natl Acad Sci USA 80:560–563
34. Burnett TS, Gallimore PH (1983) Establishment of a human keratinocyte cell line carrying complete human papillomavirus type 1 genomes: Lack of vegetative viral DNA synthesis upon keratinization. J Gen Virol 64:1509–1520
35. Duesberg PH (1983) Retroviral transforming genes in normal cells? Nature 304:219–226
36. Marcu KB (1983) Transcriptionally active c-myc oncogene is contained within NIARD, a sequence associated with chromosome translocations in B-cell neoplasia. Proc Natl Acad Sci USA 80:519–523
37. Dalla-Favera R, Martinotti S, Gallo RC (1983) Translocation and rearrangements of the c-myc oncogene locus in human undifferentiated B-cell lymphomas. Science 219:963–967
38. Yunis JJ (1983) The chromosomal basis of human neoplasia. Science 221:227–236
39. Slamon DJ, De Kernion JB, Verma IM, Clyne MJ (1984) Expression of cellular oncogenes in human malignancies. Nature 224:256–262
40. zur Hausen H (1982) Human genital cancer: synergism between two virus infections or synergism between a virus infection and initiating events? Lancet II:1370–1372
41. Boyd AL, Enquist L, Van de Woude GF, Hampar B (1981) Activation of mouse retrovirus by herpes simplex virus cloned DNA fragments. Virology 103:228–231
42. Cairns J, Logan J (1983) Cancer, step by step into carcinogenesis. Nature 304:582–583

4 · Genital Neoplasia–Papilloma Syndrome: A Unifying Concept of Human Genital Papillomavirus Infection and Expression

L.B. Twiggs, T. Okagaki, B.A. Clark, L. F. Carson, and M. Fukushima

Introduction

In the light of the increasing evidence supporting the presence of human papillomavirus (HPV) infection in human genital neoplasms, a re-evaluation of previously standard concepts of morphological categorisation and presumed biological behaviour of human genital epithelial lesions is required. Evidence of the presence of HPV in genital neoplasias has come from a variety of sources. The discovery by electron microscopy of viral-like particles in human genital condylomata was followed by their demonstration in other genital tissues [1–3]. Less strenuous ways of identifying and categorising the presence of virus were obtained by the development of antibodies to structural antigens of bovine papillomaviruses (BPV), which demonstrated BPV antigens in tissue sections by fluorescent microscopy [4–7]. The same antibodies were also used in conjunction with immunocytochemistry in the identification of papillomavirus antigens in a number of human genital lesions [8–14]. While the sensitivity of these immunological techniques may be low, particularly in demonstrating HPV in neoplastic tissues, further progress in DNA hybridisation via Southern blot techniques has allowed identification of papillomavirus DNA at an increased rate in tissue homogenates [15–23].

The identification of HPV by such techniques in multiple genital sites has led to the formulation of genital neoplasia–papilloma syndrome. This concept associates the histopathological features often seen (papillomas) with the onset of tissue proliferation (neoplasia) in multiple genital sites. In order to clarify further the role of HPV in human genital lesions, clinical features were studied in 58 patients. Results of Southern blot DNA hybridisation under low-stringency conditions were correlated with clinical history of previous and subsequent genital tract lesions.

Materials and Methods

All patients studied were referred to the Gynecologic Oncology Service at the University of Minnesota Hospitals. Tissues were excised prior to surgical removal or prior to carbon dioxide laser vaporisation and frozen in liquid nitrogen prior to DNA hybridisation. A comprehensive retrospective review of the hospital record was carried out to identify other genital tract involvement prior to and subsequent to the excision of the tissue for study.

The method used in DNA hybridisation was essentially identical to that described in our previous publications [24,25]. The frozen specimens were thawed and minced into small pieces. The tissue fragments were then suspended in 0.2 M Tris-HCl (pH 8.5), 0.1 M EDTA, 1% sodium dodecyl sulphate (SDS) containing Pronase at 500 μg/ml and incubated at 60°C for 12–24 h. The solution was cooled and potassium acetate was added to 1.43 M. After 30 min on ice, the solution was centrifuged for 20 min at 20 000 g at 4°C. The supernatant was concentrated by addition of 2 vol of ethanol. The precipitate was resuspended in 20 mM Tris-HCl (pH 7.0), 10 mM EDTA, and treated with boiled RNase at 100 μg/ml followed by incubation with SDS and Pronase, extracted with a 500 M Tris-HCl phenol–chloroform mixture of 1:1 vol/vol, and precipitated with ethanol. The samples containing HPV DNA in buffer containing 5% glycerol, 50 mM Tris acetate (pH 8.3), 2.0 mM EDTA and 1% SDS, were heated at 68°C for 10 min, and electrophoresis was carried out in 1.0% agarose gel at 60 V for 16 h.

DNA fragments were transferred from agarose gel to nitrocellulose filter with a negative pressure applied over the filter. The filters were dried at 80°C under vacuum for 2 h and hybridised under conditions of low stringency as follows: The filters were prehybridised at 37°C for 24 h in a hybridisation solution containing 500 μg/ml depurinated salmon sperm DNA, 0.1% each of bovine serum albumin, Ficoll 400 and polyvinylpyrrolidone. 20 mM sodium phosphate (pH 6.8), 1 M sodium chloride, 0.1% SDS and 30% formamide. Fresh hybridisation solution containing both nick-translated 32P-HPV-EV probe, HPV-3 related DNA isolated by Green et al. [26], and cloned Bam HI fragments (5 ng probe per ml solution; 2.5 × 10⁶ cpm/ml) and 10% dextran sulphate was added to the filters and incubated at 30°C for 20 h. Filters were washed three times in double strength SSC of pH 7.0 (single strength SSC refers to 0.15 M sodium chloride, 0.015 M sodium citrate, 0.1% SDS and 0.1% sodium pyrophosphate) at room temperature and for an additional 4 h in 3 × SSC of pH 7.0, 0.1% SDS and 0.1% sodium pyrophosphate at 40°C. Filters were dried and autoradiographed at −70°C with an intensity screen.

The patients were grouped according to their histopathological category as defined by one of the authors (T.O.). The term 'warty dysplasia' includes all patients who had dysplasia with a wart-like appearance, warty dysplasia, dysplasia with condylomatous atypia, koilocytotic dysplasia and verrucous dysplasia.

A case history is provided to illustrate in one particular patient the clinical features of the proposed genital neoplasia–papilloma syndrome.

M.C., a 36-year-old G.2, P.2, had the discovery of systemic lupus erythematosus (SLE) made in 1973, primarily due to facial erythema. At presentation renal dysfunction was noted. Treatment was begun first with prednisone and followed in 6 weeks with the addition of Immuran. Control of renal dysfunction was effected and slow reduction of the drugs was prescribed (see Fig. 4.1 for dose details). In 1977, a class IV cervical cytology led to the histopathological diagnosis of cervical intraepithelial neoplasia, grade III (carcinoma in situ). A vaginal hysterectomy was performed. In 1980 follow-up vaginal cytology was abnormal, and a colposcopic directed biopsy of a multi-focal vaginal lesion was interpreted as mild dysplasia. With electron microscopy viral-like particles 45–55 nm in diameter were seen in the superficial epithelial nuclei (Fig. 4.1). The vaginal dysplasia was successfully treated with the CO_2 laser. Recurrence of the vaginal lesion was noted in 12 months. Observation was chosen as therapy, and with the discontinuation of prednisone and Immuran and the prescribing of chloroquine, resolution of the vaginal lesions occurred.

Results

A large percentage of Southern blot hybridisations (83%) indicated the presence of HPV DNA in the varieties of genital neoplasia studied (Table 4.1). Of those tissues with negative hybridisation, two patients had genital condylomata, three patients had invasive squamous cell carcinoma (one cervix, two vulva), one patient had adenocarcinoma of the cervix, two patients had carcinoma in situ of the vulva, one patient had condylomatous carcinoma of the vulva and one patient had a cervical lymphoma.

Patients were first divided into categories correlating previous and subsequent histories of organ-specific genital lesion sites to the present abnormality; for example, single-site organ involvement, double-site organ involvement or triple-site organ involvement. A total of 23 (48%) patients had single-site organ involvement (Table 4.2). A variety of lesions were positive, ranging from condyloma of the vulva to verrucous carcinoma of the vagina, including one patient with invasive carcinoma of the vulva stage IV.

Double-site involvement with genital epithelial lesions may be classified as synchronous (occurring at the same time) or metachronous, that is, lesions developing in separate organ sites with at least a 6-month interval between the discovery of the lesions. Twelve patients (25%) had double-site involvement in both the synchronous and metachronous fashion (Tables 4.3, 4.4). Interestingly, one patient with synchronous organ involvement had verrucous carcinoma, initially treated surgically, while the recurrence of this lesion 4 years later was positive for HPV DNA. Four patients with metachronous involvement with vaginal lesions had cervical intra-epithelial neoplasia treated 4 years, 2 years and 6 months prior to the diagnosis of vaginal intra-epithelial neoplasia (Table 4.3). Metachronous double organ site involvement was seen in nine (17%) patients, three with cervix and vulva, two with vagina and vulva, and four with cervix and vagina (Tables 4.3, 4.4). Triple-site organ involvement was seen in 13 (27%)

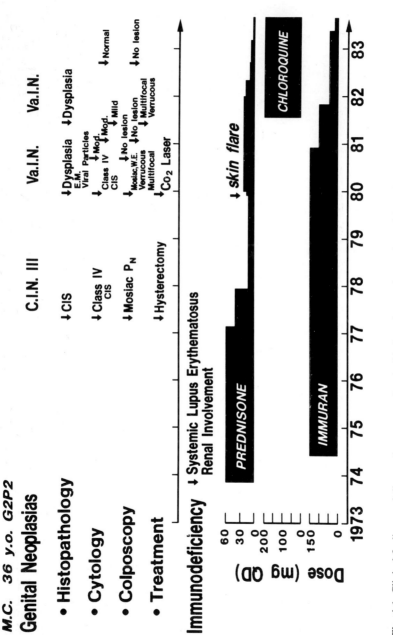

Fig. 4.1. Clinical findings and diagnostic tests correlated with drug therapy in a patient with genital neoplasia-papilloma syndrome.

Table 4.1. Histopathological categories in genital tissues excised for low-stringency Southern blot DNA hybridisation

Histopathological category	Number/percent		Number positive
Condyloma	16	(28)	14/16
Dysplasia[a,b]	23	(40)	23/23
Carcinoma in situ	11	(20	8/11
Invasive squamous			
cell carcinoma	2	(2)	0/2
Adenocarcinoma	1	(1)	0/1
Verrucous carcinoma	2	(2)	2/2
Condylomatous carcinoma	3	(5)	2/3
Lymphoma-cervix	1	(1)	0/1
Total	59		49/59

[a] Includes both dysplasia and warty dysplasia
[b] One patient had two determinations done

Table 4.2. Histopathology of the lesions in patients with single organ site involvement (cervix, vagina, vulva) and positive DNA hybridisation under low-stringency conditions

Organ involved	No. of cases	Histopathology				
		Condy-loma	Warty dysplasia	Dysplasia	Invasive carcinoma	Carcinoma in situ, Bowen's disease
Cervix	4	–	2	2	–	–
Vagina	7	–	4	2	1[a]	–
Vulva	12	3	–	–	3[b,c]	6

[a] Verrucous carcinoma with multiple recurrences
[b] One patient: condylomatous carcinoma co-existing with pseudoglandular carcinoma
[c] One patient: stage IV carcinoma S/P pelvic exenteration; NED 18 months

Table 4.3. Synchronous and metachronous double genital organ site involvement and histopathology in tissues positive by Southern blot DNA hybridisation under low-stringency conditions

Organs involved: cervix, vagina (all cases)	No. of cases 7	Histopathology			
		Condyloma	Warty dysplasia	Dysplasia	Invasive carcinoma
Synchronous only	3	–	2[a]	–	1[b]
Metachronous only	4	–	1[a,d]	3[a,c]	–

[a] Vaginal dysplasia HPV DNA positive
[b] Verrucous carcinoma originally treated surgically – recurrence positive 4 years later
[c] Three patients had hysterectomy for cervical intra-epithelial neoplasia grade III, 4 years, 2 years and 6 months
[d] Cervical intra-epithelial neoplasia grade III treated 2 years previously

Table 4.4. Metachronous double organ site involvement in tissues positive by Southern blot DNA hybridisation under low-stringency conditions

Organs involved	Histopathology		
Vagina	Condyloma		Dysplasia
Vulva	Condyloma[a]		Carcinoma in situ[a]
2	1		1
Cervix	Dysplasia		Dysplasia
Vulva	Condyloma[a]		Carcinoma in situ[a]
3	2		1

[a]   Positive site

patients, both in a metachronous and synchronous fashion (Tables 4.5, 4.6). Synchronous epithelial lesions of the cervix, vagina and vulva were associated with a number of serious systemic diseases, and patients were treated with drugs which are known to cause immunosuppression. Only one of the six patients with synchronous lesions did not have the above association. Metachronous triple-organ involvement was seen in seven patients (12%). One patient with systemic lupus erythematosus was being treated with Immuran and prednisone. Three of these patients had electron microscopic evidence for viral particles 45 to 55 nm in diameter (Fig. 4.2).

Table 4.5. Histopathology of synchronous epithelial lesions in cervix, vagina, and vulva; associated diseases and drug therapy. All patients have identification of HPV DNA by Southern blot hybridisation under low-stringency conditions

Patient	Organ–histopathology	Associate disease (drug therapy)
T.S.	Cervix–condyloma Vagina–condyloma Vulva–condyloma	Systemic lupus erythematosus (SLE) Optic neuritis Transverse myelitis (Immuran, prednisone)
K.S.	Cervix-mild dysplasia (warty) Vagina–same Vulva–condyloma	–
A.S.	Cervix–condyloma Vagina–condyloma Vulva–condylomatous carcinoma	S/P renal transplant (Immuran, prednisone)
S.H.	Cervix–mild dysplasia Vagina–moderate dysplasia Vulva–condyloma	S/P renal transplant (Immuran, prednisone)
J.S.	Cervix–condyloma Vagina–condyloma Vulva–condyloma	S/P renal transplant (Immuran, prednisone)
M.C.	Cervix–mild dysplasia Vagina–mild dysplasia Vulva–carcinoma in situ (warty)	Wegener's granulomatosis Renal failure

Table 4.6. Histopathology and date of discovery of metachronous epithelial lesions of cervix, vagina and vulva. All patients had identification of HPV DNA by Southern blot hybridisation under low-stringency conditions in at least one organ site

Patient initials	(Age)	Organ involved		
		Cervix	Vagina	Vulva
S.C.	(34)	Mild dysplasia[a] 5/82[b]	Mild dysplasia 5/82	Condyloma 1/79
B.M.	(32)	Carcinoma in situ 6/76	Severe dysplasia 6/76	Condyloma 6/72 Carcinoma in situ[a,c] 9/81
P.G.	(34)	Carcinoma in situ 12/79	Severe dysplasia[a,c] 11/80	Condyloma 3/83
L.II.	(24)	Moderate dysplasia 11/81	Condyloma[a] 6/82	Condyloma 6/82
P.L.	(41)	Carcinoma in situ 7/78	Mild dysplasia[a,c] 12/80 Condyloma 11/82	Condyloma 3/83
J.E.	(21)	Moderate dysplasia 8/80	Moderate dysplasia[a] 8/80	Condyloma 6/81
P.L.[d]	(24)	Severe dysplasia 6/75	Severe dysplasia 4/76, 7/77, 4/82	Carcinoma in situ[a] 4/81, 4/82

[a] Tissue positive
[b] Month/year of diagnosis
[c] Electron microscopy positive for viral particles
[d] SLE on Immuran and prednisone

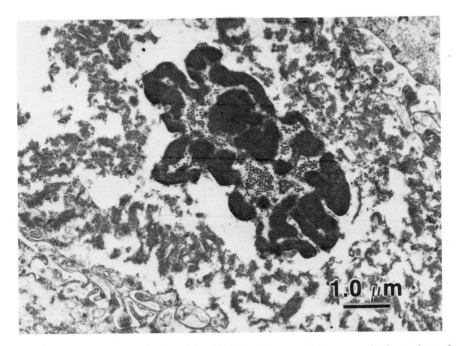

Fig. 4.2. Identification of viral particles (45–55 nm) in a crystalline array in the nucleus of warty dysplasia, positive for low stringent DNA hybridisation in the patient described (×12700).

Discussion

The ubiquity of the demonstration of human papillomavirus nucleotide sequences under low stringency Southern blot DNA hybridisation warrants further explanation. The existence of such sequences in multiple sites and types of genital tissues combined with the finding that a number of these individuals have had prior or developed subsequent genital epithelial lesions adds biological understanding to the known association of specific organ site neoplasia with other genital tract neoplasia [26–33]. This is especially cogent if one couples these observations with the hypothesis of latent viral infection. In a number of viral infections a state of latency has been demonstrated in the host cell [34,35]. Expression of the viral genome is accomplished with production of intact virus and may be accompanied by epithelial perturbations. The onset of the expression of viral DNA may be viewed as a result of a number of circumstantial associated co-factors and mechanisms which are incompletely understood (Fig. 4.3). Specifically with HPV infections viral replication is coupled with epithelial proliferation and differentiation. For example, human papillomavirus antigen demonstration via immunocytochemistry has been documented only in the terminally differentiated epithelial layers of cervical neoplastic epithelium [10–13]. Our demonstration of human papillomavirus genomes in multiple types of epithelial proliferations, ranging from benign condylomata to neoplastic lesions, is not inconsistent with the concept of latent viral expression which is coupled with epithelial proliferation. The acceptance of such a concept, however, is marred by the compartmen-

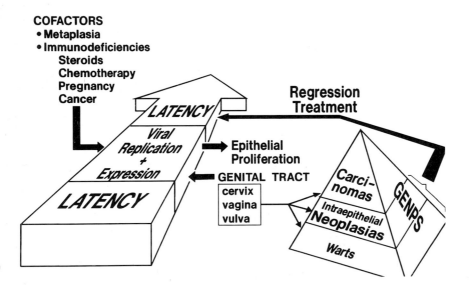

Fig. 4.3. Schematic diagram illustrating a proposed hypothesis of HPV infection and associated co-factors leading to expression of viral genome.

talising of genital tract lesions via organ sites as evidenced by the varying pathological nomenclature from organ site to site, and resultant conceptualised biological activity of the lesion dependent on its location. Our demonstration of HPV DNA in these various abnormalities warrants precise clinical correlations to pathological nomenclature in the future.

The use of Southern blot hybridisation under conditions of low stringency will certainly increase the sensitivity in the detection of viral DNA by decreasing the percentage of nucleotide homology necessary for the qualitative demonstration of viral genomes. Such a sensitive technique may lead to imprecise concepts, especially if one tacitly assumes HPV type specificity with particular histopathological categories. Past studies in dermatopathology have led to the concept of consistency of HPV type specificity in particular skin lesions using high-stringency techniques [23]. Such a concept makes the assumption that specific human papillomaviruses are causative or at least associated with specific histopathological epithelial lesions. Unfortunately, in other published data we have shown that with high-stringency Southern blot hybridisation, HPV type specificity is not consistent. For example, we have not been able to show specificity correlating HPV type to particular morphological abnormalities in vulvar, cervical and vaginal neoplasia under high stringency [24,25]. Further understanding of HPV group and type specificity to a particular lesion will depend on increasing the precision of the molecular biological characterisation of the virus and its molecular constituents.

The susceptibility to viral infection in patients known to be immunocompromised is a known fact, and studies noting the development of multiple types of epithelial abnormalities, including an occasional carcinoma of the skin associated with immunosuppression have been published [36,37,38]. In this investigation the finding of increased numbers of patients with metachronous site involvement with immunodysfunction (Fig. 4.4), defined as patients with rheumatoid diseases or patients treated with immunosuppressive drugs, adds credence to the hypothesis that such patients have had previous HPV infections and during a period of immunological disturbance, the latent viral genome is expressed and epithelial proliferations with intact virions are demonstrated.

Before accepting that these epithelial proliferations are expressions of latent viral infections, a number of facts must be specified, as has been outlined by Rivers and Evans [39,40]. Immunological demonstration of causation of viral

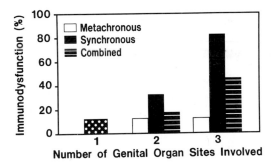

Fig. 4.4. Percentage of patients with immunodysfunction relative to synchronous and metachronous occurrence of genital lesions.

infection has as a prerequisite to illness a regular absence of viral specific antibody. In HPV infections such investigations have not been carried out. Also, regular antibody appearance during illness, coupled with antibody production, must be accompanied temporarily by the presence of viruses in appropriate tissues. Baird, measuring serum antibodies to bovine papillomavirus antigens, has shown that patients with various epithelial proliferations, including cervical cancer, have a higher incidence of circulating antibodies than patients used as controls [41]. This is the first step towards regular associations and immunological proof of viral infection. Furthermore it is important, as Rivers and Evans indicated, to show that the absence of antibodies indicates immunity, and as such the production of antibody (immunisation) prevents disease [39,40]. Such ongoing studies will need to fulfil these criteria before one can accept the concept that HPV is causative of the lesions with which it is associated.

Summary

In summary, tissues from 58 patients with epithelial lesions of the genital tract were studied by low-stringency Southern blot DNA hybridisation. A large number of patients with multiple synchronous genital tract sites of epithelial proliferation were noted to have a high incidence of immunological dysfunction. Evidence presented here is consistent with the concept that a latent human papillomavirus infection is both associated with and causative of neoplastic genital tract proliferations. A descriptive term to associate genital neoplastic papillomatous lesions known to contain HPV has been coined, genital neoplasia–papilloma syndrome.

References

1. Charles A (1960) Electron microscope observations on the human wart. Dermatologica 121:193–203
2. Almeida JD, Howatson AF, Williams MG (1962) Electron microscope study of human warts; sites of virus production and nature of inclusion bodies. J Invest Dermatol 38:337–345
3. Dunn AEG, Ogilvie MM (1968) Intranuclear virus particles in human genital wart tissue: observations on the ultrastructure of the epidermal layer, J Ultrastructure Res 22:282–295
4. Pass F, Janis R, Marcus DM (1970) Antigens of human wart tissue. J Invest Dermatol 56:305–310
5. Pyrhonen S, Penttinen K (1972) Wart-virus antibodies and the prognosis of wart disease. Lancet II:1330–1332
6. Jensen AB, Rosenthal JD, Olson C, Pass F, Lancaster WD, Shah K, (1980) Immunological relatedness of papillomaviruses from different species. J Natl Cancer Inst 64:495–500
7. Dunn J, Weinstein L, Droegemueller W, Meinke W (1981) Immunologic detection of condylomata accuminata-specific antigens. Obstet Gynecol 57:351–356
8. Woodruff JD, Braun L, Cavalieri R, Gupta P, Pass F, Shah KV (1980) Immunologic identification of papillomavirus antigen in condyloma tissues from the female genital tract. Obstet Gynecol 56:727–732
9. Ferenczy A, Braun L, Shah KV (1981) Human papillomavirus (HPV) in condylomatous lesions of the cervix. A comparative ultrastructural and immunohistochemical study. Am J Surg Pathol 5:661–670
10. Kurman RJ, Shah KH, Lancaster WD, Jenson AB (1981) Immunoperoxidase localization of

papillomavirus antigens in cervical dysplasia and vulvar condylomas. Am J Obstet Gyncol 140:931–935

11. Kurman RJ, Sanz LE, Jenson AB, Perry S, Lancaster WD, (1982) Papillomavirus infection of the cervix. I. Correlation of histology with viral structural antigens and DNA sequences. Int J Gynecol Pathol 1:17–28

12. Syrjanen KJ, Pyrhonen S (1982) Demonstration of human papillomavirus antigen in the condylomatous lesions of the uterine cervix by immunoperoxidase technique. Gynecol Obstet Invest 14:90–96

13. Kurman RJ, Jenson AB, Lancaster WD (1983) Papillomavirus infection of the cervix. II. Relationship to intraepiethelial neoplasia based on the presence of specific viral structural proteins. Am J Surg Pathol 7:39–52

14. Southern EM (1975) Detection of specific sequences among DNA fragments separated by gel electrophoresis. J Mol Biol 98:503–520

15. zur Hausen H (1976) Condylomata accuminata and human genital cancer. Cancer Res 36:794–796

16. Orth G, Favre M, Jablonska S, Brylak K, Croissant O (1978) Viral sequences related to a human skin papillomavirus in genital warts. Nature 275:334–336

17. Law MF, Lancaster WD, Howley PM (1979) Conserved polynucleotide sequences among the genomes of papillomaviruses. J Virol 32:199–207

18. Howley PM, Israel MA, Law MF, Martin MA (1979) A rapid method for detecting and mapping homology between heterologous DNA: evaluation of polyomavirus genomes. J Biol Chem 254:4876–4883

19. Favre M, Orth G, Croissant O, Yaniv M (1975) Human papillomavirus DNA: physical map. Proc Natl Acad Sci USA 72:4810–4814

20. Gissmann L, zur Hausen H (1976) Human papillomaviruses DNA: physical mapping and genetic heterogeneity. Proc Natl Acad Sci USA 73:1310–1313

21. Orth G, Favre M, Croissant O (1977) Characterization of a new type of human papillomavirus that causes skin warts. J Virol 24:108–120

22. Gissmann L, Pfister H, zur Hausen H (1977) Human papillomavirus (HPV): characterization of four different isolates. Virology 76:569–580

23. Orth G, Jablonska S, Favre M, Croissant O, Jarzabek-Chorzelska M, Rzesa G (1978) Characterization of two types of human papillomaviruses in lesions of epidermodysplasia verruciformis. Proc Natl Acad Sci USA 75:1537–1541

24. Okagaki T, Twiggs LB, Zachow KR, Clark BA, Ostrow RS, Faras AJ (1983) Identification of human papillomavirus DNA in cervical and vaginal intraepithelial neoplasia with molecular cloned virus-specific DNA probe. Int J Gynecol Pathol 2:153–159

25. Twiggs LB, Okagaki T, Zachow KR, Clark BA, Ostrow RS. Faras AK (to be published) Identification of human papillomavirus DNA in vulvar intra-epithelial neoplasia with molecular cloned virus-specific DNA probe.

26. Green M, Brackmann KH, Sanders PR, Loewenstein PM, Freel JH, Eisinger M, Switlyk SA (1982) Isolation of a human papillomavirus from a patient with epidermodysplasia verruciformis: Presence of related viral DNA genomes in human urogenital tumors. Proc Natl Acad Sci USA, 79:4441–4443

27. Newman W, Cromer SK (1959) The multicentric origin of the female anogenital tract. Surg Gynecol and Obstet 108:273–276

28. Jimerson GK, Merrill JA (1970) Multicentric squamous malignancy involving both the cervix and vulva. Cancer 26:150–156

29. Rutledge F, Sinclair M (1968) Treatment of intraepithelial carcinoma of the vulva by skin incision and graft. Am J Obstet Gynecol 102:806–815

30. Collins CG, Kushner J, Lewis GN, LaPoint R (1955) Noninvasive malignancy of the vulva. Obstet Gynecol 6:339–347

31. Boutselis JG (1972) Intraepithelial carcinoma of the vulva. Am J Obstet Gynecol 113:733–740

32. Woodruff JD, Julian C, Puray T, Mermut S, Katayama P (1973) The contemporary challenge of carcinoma in situ of the vulva. Am J Obstet Gynecol 115:677–684

33. Friedrich G, Wilkenson EJ, Fu YS (1980) Carcinoma in situ of the vulva, a continuing challenge. Am J Obstet Gynecol 136:830–841

34. Kunshner A, Kandour AI, David B (1978) Early vulva carcinoma. Am J Obstet Gynecol 132:599–606

35. Baringer JR (1975) Herpes simplex virus infection of nervous tissue in animals and man. Prog Med Virol 20:1–4

36 Black FL, Hierholzer WJ, Pinheiro FP et al. (1974) Evidence for persistence of infectious agents in isolated human populations. Am J Epidemiol 100(3):230–232

37. Seski JC, Reinhalter ER, Silva J (1978) Abnormalities of the lymphocyte transformation in women with condyloma acuminata. Obstet Gynecol 55:188–196
38. Westburg SP, Stone OJ (1973) Multiple cutaneous squamous cell carcinomas during immunosuppressive therapy. Arch Dermatol 107:893–896
39. Rivers TM (1937) Viruses and Koch's postulates. J Bacteriol 33:1–25
40. Evans AS (1976) Causation and disease: the Henle–Koch postulates revisited. Yale J Biol Med 49:175–188
41. Baird PJ (1983) Serological evidence for the association of papillomavirus infection and cervical neoplasia. Lancet II:17–18

5 · Cervical Cancer Screening — Revisions of the Walton Report*

J.A. Carmichael

Introduction

In 1967 a National Health Care Programme was established in Canada which provided total health and hospital care for every citizen of the country. With the exception of annual premiums in the Provinces of British Columbia, Alberta and Ontario (premiums which only minimally contributed to the cost) funding for the programme was generated through general taxation at the Provincial and Federal levels. This health care programme entitles any citizen at any time to see any physician for any reason and as often as he or she feels necessary. While funding is by general taxation, payment to the physician remains on a fee for service basis. Despite warnings from the Medical Associations, both at the Federal and Provincial levels, the plan was introduced with the cost results shown in Fig. 5.1.

As a result of the initial staggering rise in costs of health care, a number of Task Forces were instituted by the Federal government to review health care programmes currently in existence in order to determine their efficacy and to justify their costs. One such was the Task Force on 'Cervical Cancer Screening Programs'.

The observations and recommendations developed by the initial Task Force— the so-called Walton Report of 1976—are briefly reviewed in this chapter, as are some of the implications of this report and, finally, the observations and recommendations of the re-convened Federal Task Force on cervical screening [2,4] which made its final report in October 1982.

* The figures published in this report are used with the permission of the Department of National Health and Welfare of Canada.

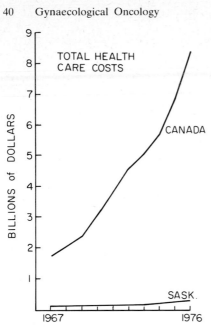

Fig. 5.1. Total health care costs in Canada since the National Health Care Program was established in 1967.

Existing Data

The members of the Federal Task Force agreed at the outset that invasive squamous carcinoma of the cervix is preceded by a series of progressively abnormal premalignant changes, i.e. dysplasia and carcinoma in situ. They also agreed that these dysplastic and in situ changes could be accurately detected by cervical cytological smears.

The duration of this pre-invasive phase, rate and frequency of progression from one dysplastic level to another, and the rate and frequency of regression were unknown. On the basis of the British Columbia screening programme experience, it appeared that the peak age for pre-invasive disease was in the middle 20s and for invasive disease the middle to late 50s, suggesting a period of pre-invasive change as long as 15–20 years.

A great deal has been written about the epidemiology of carcinoma of the cervix. Despite a number of recognised and associated factors the two consistent epidemiological observations associated with carcinoma of the cervix are (1) onset of intercourse at an early age, and (2) intercourse with multiple partners. The Task Force acknowledged certain aetiological observations including herpes simplex virus II, human papilloma virus, and the male factor. The exact role of these associated factors at the time of publication of the initial Task Force report was (and still is) uncertain.

Both the mortality and incidence of carcinoma of the cervix vary considerably throughout the world, and indeed in Canada from Province to Province (Tables 5.1 and 5.2). On the basis of Canadian data the Task Force was able to identify an indirect relationship between cervical screening activity and mortality from car-

Table 5.1. Mortality from carcinoma of the uterus, 1965–1969

Country	Mortality[a]	Country	Mortality[a]
Israel	9.5	Yugoslavia	24.0
Philippines	11.4	Czechoslovakia	24.8
Greece	12.6	Portugal	25.4
Bulgaria	14.3	Japan	25.9
Australia	15.8	Hong Kong	26.9
Eire	16.8	Italy	26.9
New Zealand	18.2	West Germany	27.1
Northern Ireland	18.4	Singapore	28.8
Norway	18.5	Panama	28.9
Finland	18.9	Taiwan	33.8
Canada	19.1	Poland	35.2
Sweden	19.8	Denmark	35.5
United States	19.8	Hungary	35.5
Netherlands	20.3	Mauritius	35.7
Switzerland	20.7	Austria	36.3
England and Wales	20.7	Mexico	39.1
Scotland	21.2	Chile	43.7
France	22.1	Romania	45.5
Belgium	22.8		

[a]   Age-standardised rates per 100 000 women aged 35 to 64.

cinoma of the cervix throughout the various regions of the country (Fig. 5.2). Unfortunately a similar beneficial relationship between screening activity and incidence of carcinoma of the cervix from community to community in Canada could not demonstrated.

A dramatic relationship between screening activities and falling incidence of carcinoma of the cervix is seen in the Province of British Columbia (Fig. 5.3). This is probably the oldest and largest screening programme available with accurate figures, and is certainly the 'flagship' for screening programmes in Canada. This convincing relationship could not be confirmed when the experiences of other provinces were reviewed. In Alberta, which had a registry for invasive carcinoma for some 10 years prior to the introduction of a screening programme, it can be quite clearly shown that the fall in incidence of carcinoma of the cervix was well established prior to the introduction of such a cervical cytological screening programme (Fig. 5.4). This can also be demonstrated for the province of

Table 5.2. Incidence of invasive carcinoma of the cervix (ICD 180), Canada, 1969–72

Province	Incidence[a]
Newfoundland	53.3
Prince Edward Island	54.5
Nova Scotia	54.1
New Brunswick	51.1
Quebec	32.9
Ontario	55.1[b]
Manitoba	37.3
Saskatchewan	22.5
Alberta	29.1
British Columbia	39.3

[a]   Age-standardised rates per 100 000 women aged 35 to 64.
[b]   Data from 1966 Ontario cancer incidence survey.

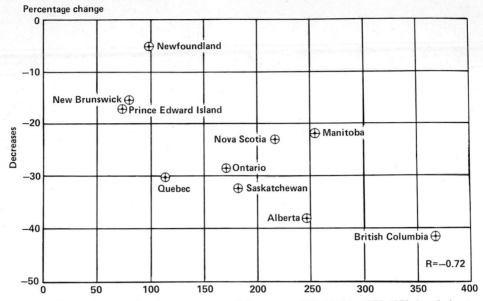

Fig. 5.2. Change in mortality from carcinoma of the uterus, 1960–1962 to 1970–1972, in relation to screening rate in 1966 (based on 3-year average age-standardised truncated mortality rates per 100 000 women aged 30–64. Sources: Statistics Canada and surveys of the Canadian Society of Cytology).

Saskatchewan (Fig. 5.5). Review of screening programmes in other countries was equally unconvincing. The Task Force was therefore unable to assume a relationship between cervical screening and incidence of invasive carcinoma of the cervix.

Recommendations for Screening Programmes

A considerable amount of attention was devoted in the Task Force report to the philosophy and development of successful screening programmes, training requirements for cytotechnicians and cytopathologists, quality control of cytological laboratories, etc. A number of recommendations were made by the Task Force; these dealt with the maintenance and surveillance of quality of cervical cytological laboratories, appropriate follow-up mechanisms for patients who have been identified as having abnormal cytological smears, and appropriate and universal terminology for reporting purposes from one province to the other. Details are given in the original publication [1].

The most publicised and controversial recommendation made by the Federal Task Force was related to the periodicity of a cervical screening programme. The Task Force recommended that any woman who has ever been coitally active should have a cervical smear at the onset of her coital activity and this should be repeated within 1 year—to minimise the risk of false negative reports. Thereafter, until the age of 35, a cervical smear should taken once every 3 years, and from 35

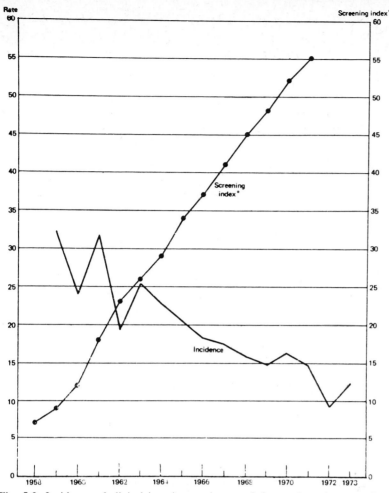

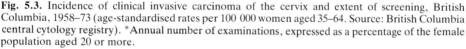

Fig. 5.3. Incidence of clinical invasive carcinoma of the cervix and extent of screening, British Columbia, 1958–73 (age-standardised rates per 100 000 women aged 35–64. Source: British Columbia central cytology registry). *Annual number of examinations, expressed as a percentage of the female population aged 20 or more.

to 60 once every 5 years. Should a patient reach 60 years of age with a history of repeated negative cytology she should be dropped from a screening programme.

The Task Force identified a sub-group of people at risk to be termed 'high risk'. These women should be screened annually. This group would include those young women who began intercourse at an early age and with multiple partners, those who had entered into an unstable sexual relationship, and those who had a history of genital infection such as herpes simplex virus II, human papilloma virus or any other circumstance identified by her physician which might place her in a high-risk group.

In Canada cervical screening is universally available but is on a voluntary basis. As with other voluntary health care programmes, it is the high-risk group that has

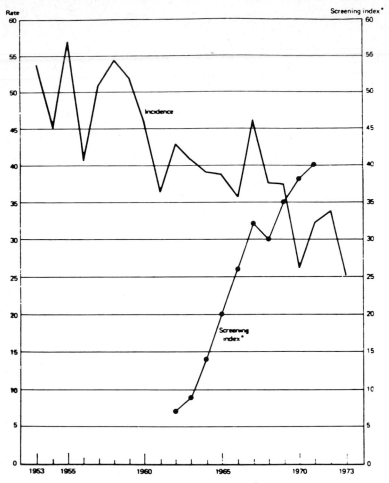

Fig. 5.4. Incidence of carcinoma of the cervix and extent of screening, Alberta, 1953–73 (age-standardised rates per 100 000 women aged 35–64. Source: Alberta provincial cancer registry). *Annual number of examinations, expressed as a percentage of the female population aged 20 or more.

tended to be omitted from the screening programmes to date. It was the Task Force's opinion that by stopping annual cervical cytological examinations for the 'at risk' group and encouraging high-risk groups to enter a screening programme, a rational universal total population screening programme could be supported by the cytological laboratory facilities currently in operation in the country.

Reactions to the Walton Report

The Task Force report was favourably received by most health care organisations, planners and Public Health authorities throughout the world. Its recommendations were incorporated into teaching programmes at most medical schools in

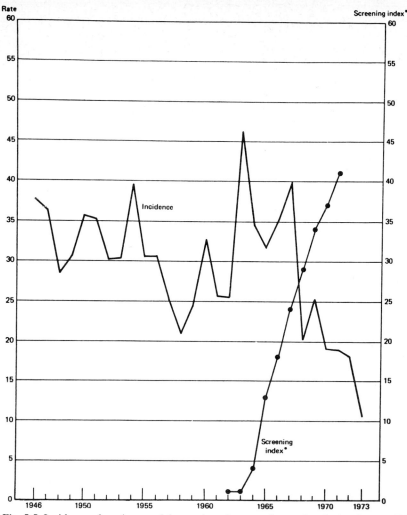

Fig. 5.5. Incidence of carcinoma of the cervix and extent of screening, Saskatchewan, 1946–1973 (age-standardised incidence rates per 100 000 women aged 35–64. Source: Saskatchewan Cancer Commission). *Annual number of examinations, expressed as a percentage of the female population aged 20 or more.

Canada. The report was received with less than overwhelming enthusiasm by the practising physicians of the country. There was no significant decrease in the frequency of cervical screening nor any significant increase in the percentage of the total population covered. Furthermore, little or nothing was done by government authorities regarding the establishment of cytological registries or follow-up programmes, or for quality control of cervical cytological laboratories.

Partly because of this lack of response and partly because of new information that had become available, particularly from the British Columbia cohorts study [3] which enabled the development of certain patient mathematical models, the Federal Task Force on cervical screening was reconvened at the request of the

Federal government. The results of this Task Force were published in October 1982 [2,4].

Results of the Reconvened Study

The British Columbia cohorts study, while not able to define exactly the frequency and rate of progression and regression of the various degrees of pre-invasive change, did allow a better understanding of the natural history of pre-invasive disease and provided the observation that approximately 60% of patients with in situ carcinoma of the cervix will progress to invasive disease if left untreated. Mathematical models based on the B.C. cohort study provided accurate estimations of the effect of various screening schedules on the mortality and incidence of carcinoma of the cervix (Fig. 5.6, Table 5.3). Mathematical models

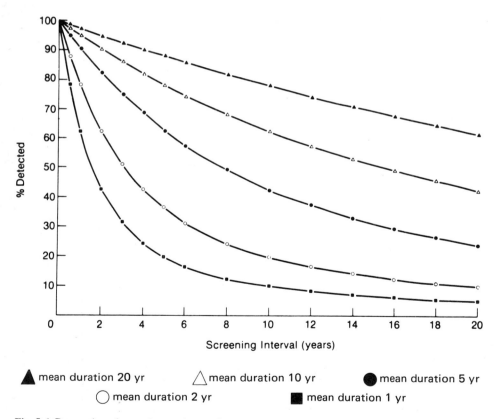

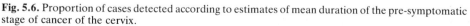

Fig. 5.6. Proportion of cases detected according to estimates of mean duration of the pre-symptomatic stage of cancer of the cervix.

Table 5.3. Results of computer simulation screening programs.

Starting age	Frequency (years)	Total tests	Mortality per 10^4	Reduction (%)
At risk				
20	3–5	11	7.8	93
High risk				
20	3–5	11	11.0	92
20	1–5	21	1.3	99

are understandably viewed with some caution by the practising physicians; how-ever, they do provide a guide to the development of practical screening programmes.

Two additional very important observations were made by the reconvened Task Force. First, the incidence of carcinoma of the cervix in Canada was no longer decreasing and indeed was showing a subtle but definite rise. This increase in incidence was seen almost exclusively in the younger age groups (Figs. 5.7, 5.8). Secondly, recent reports from the Scandinavian countries demonstrated a

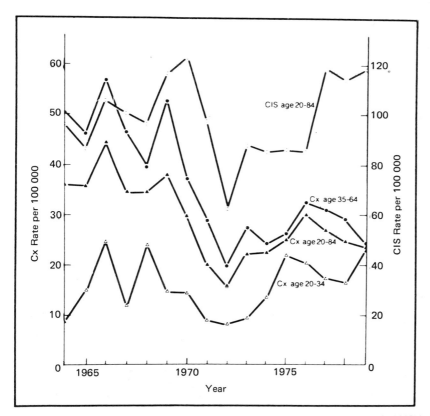

Fig. 5.7. Incidence of cancer of the cervix *(Cx)* and of carcinoma in situ of the cervix *(CIS)* in Manitoba. 1964–1979, age standardised rates per 100 000.

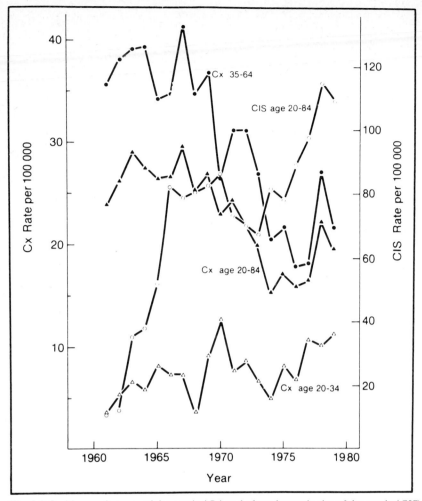

Fig. 5.8. Incidence of cancer of the cervix (*Cx*) and of carcinoma in situ of the cervix (*CIS*) in Alberta, 1961–1979, age standardised rates per 100 000.

reduced incidence of carcinoma of the cervix in those countries that had introduced a screening programme, i.e. Iceland, Denmark, Sweden and Finland, all of whom introduced screening programmes in the mid 1960s. The single exception was Norway, which decided not to introduce a screening programme and did not experience a fall in the incidence of carcinoma of the cervix (Fig. 5.9). This appears to have put the final nail in the coffin of the argument regarding the ability of a cervical screening programme to reduce the incidence of invasive squamous carcinoma of the cervix. It should be noted that these screening programmes achieve their results with screening frequencies of 3 or 5 years.

The recommendations of the reconvened Federal Task Force on cervical screening were, in a large part, similar to the original Task Force report. For

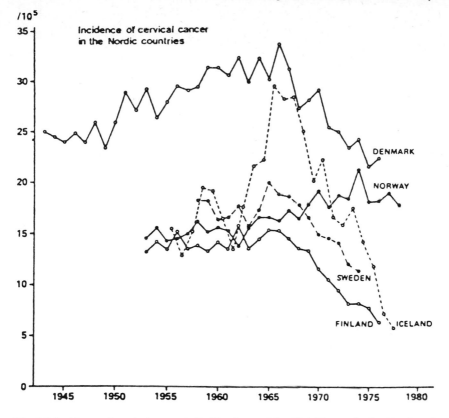

Fig. 5.9. Incidence of cervical cancer in the Nordic countries. Only Norway had not instituted a cervical cancer screening programme.

details the reader is referred again to the original texts [1,2,4]. The most significant recommendation was a change in the periodicity of screening as follows: all patients who have ever been sexually active under the age of 35 should be screened on an annual basis. It was the opinion of the Task Force that in 1982 most women in Canada under the age of 35 would have entered into their coital activity after the mid 1960s. If our understanding of the epidemiology of carcinoma of the cervix is correct and if we correctly comprehend the changing sexual mores of our society, then for practical purposes in terms of a screening programme all women under the age of 35 should be considered high risk and therefore screened annually.

It was again demonstrated by the reconvened Federal Task Force that the overwhelming majority of patients identified with pre-invasive changes are under the age of 35. On this basis the change from annual to five-year screening was set at 35 years of age. The remaining screening schedules remain as stated in the original report.

References

1. Blanchet M, Boyes DA, Carmichael JA, Marshall KG, Miller AB, Thompson DW, Walton RJ (1976) Cervical Cancer Screening Programs (The Walton Report). Can Med Assoc J 114:1003–1031
2. Allen HH, Anderson GH, Boyes DA et al. (1982) Cervical Cancer Screening Program, Summary of 1982 Canadian Task Force Report. Can Med Assoc J 127:581–589
3. Boyes DA, Morrison B, Knox EG, Draper GJ, Miller AB (1982) A Cohort Study of Cervical Cancer Screening in British Columbia. Clin Invest Med 5:1–29
4. Allen HH, Anderson GH, Boyes DA et al. (1982) Cervical Cancer Screening Program, 1982. Ministry of National Health and Welfare, Ottawa, Canada

6 · The Influence of Colposcopy on Cone Biopsy Practice

P.M. Lenehan, G.S. Sykes, H.B. Morris and M.F. Charnock

Introduction

The use of colposcopy is recognised to be an important part of the evaluation of the woman with an abnormal cervical smear [1]. Its use, with colposcopically directed punch biopsy, has meant that many women who would have had cone biopsies in the past can now be effectively treated by methods of local destruction. Cone biopsy is reserved for women with lesions assessed as unsuitable for local destruction.

Following the appointment of two trained colposcopists in February 1981 at the John Radcliffe Hospital, Oxford, it was possible to establish in Oxford a regular colposcopy service available for the assessment of all patients with abnormal cervical cytology. This also meant an increased reliance on local destruction of cervical intra-epithelial neoplasia (CIN) in suitable cases. While the effect of this has been a reduction in the proportion of cases of CIN managed by cone biopsy, it was not known whether the dimensions of those cone biopsy specimens now excised differed significantly from those excised in the years before the colposcopy service was introduced. This was assessed retrospectively by comparing the features of cone biopsy specimens excised in two 12-month periods—one before and one after the introduction of the colposcopy service.

Methodology

The pathology reports of all cone biopsy specimens excised in the periods 1 January 1976 to 31 December 1976 and 1 April 1981 to 31 March 1982 were compared retrospectively. The dimensions, and details about completeness of excision of lesion, were noted. The slides of all specimens incompletely reported in the two periods were examined by one of us (H.B.M.). If the lesion extended to the cut edge of the specimen it was considered incompletely excised. Case notes of patients with incomplete excision of lesions were reviewed for information about further management.

In both periods cone biopsy excisions were done by the registrars, senior registrars and consultants on regular operating lists. Prior to excision, lesions were delineated by Lugol's iodine stain. In the 1981/82 period colpodiagrams and colposcopic assessment notes informed the surgeon about the location and extent of the lesion and so helped him to decide the most suitable dimensions of the cone biopsy. In 1981/82 all colposcopic assessments were done by the two trained colposcopists within 1 month of cone biopsy. In 1976 the few colposcopic assessments that were done were by different doctors of varying expertise in colposcopy.

Results

While there were similar numbers of cone biopsy excisions in 1976 and the 1981/82 period (Table 6.1), the proportion of women with positive cytology managed by cone biopsy excision was significantly greater in 1976 (76/106) than in 1981/82 (71/246) ($\chi^2 = 109$, 1 df, $P < 0.001$). In 1976 and 1981/82 cone biopsies were compared by subgrouping of specimens into 5 mm intervals of depth and diameter of base

Table 6.1. Comparison of the incidence and features of incomplete excision cone biopsies in 1976 and the 1981/82 period

	1976		1981/82	
	n	%	n	%
Number of patients undergoing cone biopsy	76		70	
Complete excision	59	77.6	49	70.0
Incomplete excision	17	22.4	21	30.0
Margin involved with incomplete excision				
Ectocervical	7	9.2	5	7.1
Endocervical	7	9.2	12	17.1
Both	3	3.9	4	5.7
Depth of cone with incompletely excised lesion at endocervical margin				
≤ 2 cm	9	11.8	11	15.7
> 2 cm	1	1.3	5	7.1

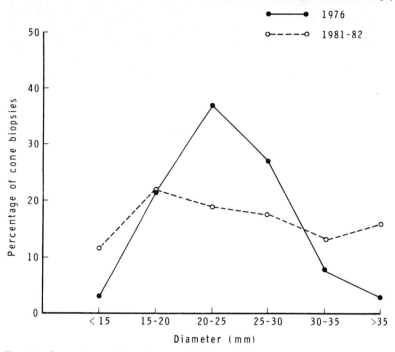

Fig. 6.1. Comparison of the diameter of the base of cone biopsies in 1976 and the 1981/82 period.

(Figs. 6.1, 6.2). There were significant differences in both dimension measurements between the two records (depth: $\chi^2 = 43.15$, 5 df, $P < 0.001$; diameter : $\chi^2 = 15.42$, 5 df, $0.001 < P < 0.01$). The cone biopsies excised in 1981/82 tended to be deeper and of more varied diameters than those excised in 1976. The age (mean ± 1SD) of the patients who had cone biopsies in 1976 (34.74 ± 9.13) and in the 1981/82 period (36.29 ± 10.64) did not differ significantly (student's t–test). Twelve of the patients with positive smears in 1976 (11.2%) and 198 (80.5%) in the 1981/82 period had colposcopic assessments.

In Table 6.1 the details of completeness of excision of lesions in the two periods are presented. Incomplete excision was more frequent in the 1981/82 period (30.0% of cases) than in 1976 (22.4% of cases) although the difference was not statistically significant (chi squared analysis).

Of the patients with incomplete excision of their disease, two in 1976 and one in the 1981/82 period were diagnosed as having invasive carcinoma. Two patients in each series with incompletely excised lesions were lost to follow-up. Awareness of incomplete excision of CIN prompted further treatment in three patients in 1976: either hysterectomy (two patients), without subsequent evidence of residual disease in the specimens, or electrodiathermy (one patient). The other ten patients have been followed by regular cervical cytology, which to date has been negative in nine cases and positive in one. This patient had negative cytology until 1982, when the diagnosis of invasive carcinoma of the cervix stage IIB was made following a positive smear. Twelve patients from the 1981/82 period have had further treatment: either hysterectomy (11 patients), with residual CIN found in

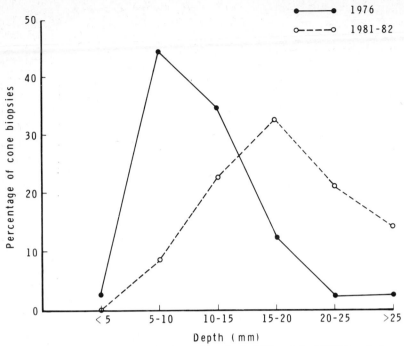

Fig. 6.2. Comparison of the depth of cone biopsies in 1976 and the 1981/82 period.

four specimens only, or repeat cone biopsy (one patient), without residual disease. The other six patients have been followed up for a minimum of 1 year by cervical cytology and colposcopic assessment. This has been negative in five cases and positive for one who has been diagnosed as having residual CIN. Thus, from the two series, only one patient with incompletely excised CIN has subsequently developed invasive carcinoma. A high proportion, 12 of 13 (92.3%) in 1976 and 13 of 18 (72.2%) in the 1981/82 period, have not had residual or recurrent CIN.

Discussion

The trend towards deeper cone biopsies and those of more varied diameters excised in the period following the introduction of the colposcopy service was probably due to the surgeon's aim of tailoring the shape of the cone biopsy specimen to the area of abnormality on the cervix. Furthermore, cone biopsy excision was done largely in cases unsuitable for treatment by local destruction. This was in contrast to the practice in 1976, when most cone biopsies were not subsequent to colposcopy. Therefore, it was of concern that colposcopic assessment had not made a significant impact on the completeness of excision of lesion. Incomplete excision at the ectocervical margin still occurred in spite of Lugol's iodine stain. This may have resulted from many different surgeons doing the operations and the colposcopic assessment having been undertaken days prior to cone biopsy. This practice is likely to be followed by many centres in the United Kingdom. Incomplete excision of a lesion at the ectocervical margin should not pose the same problems at follow-up as incomplete excision at the endocervical margin. The ectocervix is more assessable by colposcopic examination and cytology. Colposcopy is of no use in assessing the depth of a lesion extending into the endocervical canal beyond view. The surgeon had been advised in these cases to excise deep cone biopsy specimens. Even after pre-operative colposcopic assessment, incomplete excision at the endocervical margin occurred in 16 out of 70 cases (22.8%), and 5 (31.3%) of these were in spite of a specimen whose depth was greater than 2 cm. It was only when the depth of the endocervical canal exceeded 2.5 cm that the margins of all such specimens were free of disease.

Much of the immediate and long-term morbidity associated with cone biopsy [2] is likely to be increased by deeper excisions [3,4]. Contact hysteroscopy may be of use in these cases to visualise the entire extent of a lesion extending into the endocervical canal [5,6]. Using the Hamou microcolpohysteroscope in 13 patients, Soutter et al. recently demonstrated a good correlation between their measurements and those found on subsequent histological examination [7].

It was reassuring that only one (3.2%) of the 35 patients with incompletely excised CIN lesions subsequently had invasive carcinoma. The large number of patients without evidence of residual CIN at repeat cone biopsy or hysterectomy may be due to tissue necrosis or inflammation at the surgical margins resulting in the destruction of residual disease. This would imply that such further *immediate* surgical procedures with associated potential problems are *not* always justified. Careful follow-up with both cytology and colposcopy may be adequate, especially in those patients wishing to use their reproductive potential after the surgery.

Acknowledgements. We are indebted to Dr. A. Spriggs, Cytology Department, Churchill Hospital, Oxford, for providing the facilities for extracting patient data, and to Mrs P. Yudkin, Nuffield Department of Obstetrics, for assistance with the statistical analysis.

References

1. Sharp F, Jordan JA (1982) How many colposcopy centres do we need in the UK? In: Jordan JA, Sharp F, Singer A (eds) Preclinical neoplasia of the cervix. Proceedings of the Study Group, RCOG, London, pp 281–286
2. Jones JM, Sweetman P, Hibbard BM (1979) The outcome of pregnancy after cone biopsy of the cervix: A case control study. Br J Obstet Gynaecol 86:913–916
3. McCrum A, Leusley DM, Terry PB, Emens JM, Jordan JA (1983) Cone biopsy of the cervix: The influence of cone dimensions on complications. Summaries, 23rd British Congress of Obstetrics and Gynaecology, Summary 106, p 115
4. Leiman G, Harrison NA, Rubin A (1980) Pregnancy following conisation of the cervix: Complications related to cone size. Am J Obstet Gynaecol 136:14–18
5. Soutter WP, Fenton DW, Gudgeon P, Sharp F (1983) Microcolpohysteroscopic evaluation of the extent of endocervical involvement by cervical intraepithelial neoplasia. Summaries, 23rd British Congress of Obstetrics and Gynaecology, Summary 105, p 114
6. Baggish MS, Dorsey JH (1982) Contact hysteroscopic evaluation of the endocervix as an adjunct to colposcopy. Obstet Gynaecol 60:107–110

7. Soutter WP, Fenton DW, Gudgeon P, Sharp F (1984) Quantitative microcolpohysteroscopic evaluation of the extent of endocervical involvement by cervical intraepithelial neoplasia. Br J Obstet Gynaecol 91:712

7 · Micro-invasive Carcinoma of the Cervix: A Follow-up Study of 561 Cases

P. Kolstad and T. Iversen

Introduction

Mestwerdt in 1947 [1] defined microcarcinoma of the cervix as a lesion which infiltrated less than 5 mm into the stroma. At the Norwegian Radium Hospital we have used this definition since the early 1950s and in our studies allocated all cases within this group to stage Ia. The first report from our institution on diagnosis and treatment of stage Ia carcinoma of the cervix was published in 1969 [2]. The material comprised a total of 177 cases, 164 of which were squamous cell carcinomas. The patients were followed-up for 5–17 years. In four cases metastases to the pelvic wall were detected; however, the review disclosed that two of these should probably have been classified as stage Ib because there were insufficient data to evaluate the true extent of invasion. It was concluded that a diagnosis of microcarcinoma should preferably be made on a conisation specimen. The risk of spread in stage Ia was found to be so small that routine treatment of the pelvic lymph nodes with lymphadenectomy or irradiation should not be necessary.

The second study from our hospital on stage Ia carcinoma of the cervix appeared 10 years later in 1979 [3]. This time the aim was to evaluate the significance of depth of infiltration and the occurrence of vessel (capillary-like space, endothelial-lined space) involvement. A total of 122 patients in whom, during the primary operation, all pathological tissue was removed and examined microscopically, were followed-up for 5–25 years. Vessel invasion was found in 2 out of 67 cases with depth of infiltration less than 1 mm, compared with 12 out of 55 cases with infiltration of 1–5 mm. Spread to the pelvic wall was detected during follow-up in 1 of 108 cases with no capillary-space involvement, in none of 6 cases with questionable involvement and in 3 of 8 with unquestionable involvement. Of the 4 cases with lymph node metastases, 3 were found more than 5 years after primary treatment, the last one after a follow-up period of 13 years.

The aim of the present study is to clarify whether the treatment protocol introduced in the early 1970s is adequate, too conservative, or too radical.

Material

Altogether, 969 cases of carcinoma of the cervix were classified as stage Ia during the years 1951–1980 (Fig. 7.1). Of these, 561 patients were treated in the years 1971–1980. Histological diagnoses are shown in Table 7.1. Squamous cell carcinoma was found in 533 cases.

Age distribution is illustrated in Fig. 7.2. The majority of the patients were between 30 and 50 years of age; the youngest was 21 and the oldest 79. Mean age was 45.7 years: this is 4 years older than patients with cervical intra-epithelial neoplasia and 4 years younger than patients with stage Ib lesions (Fig. 7.3). The data in Fig. 7.3 are based upon a total of 3474 patients with cervical cancer.

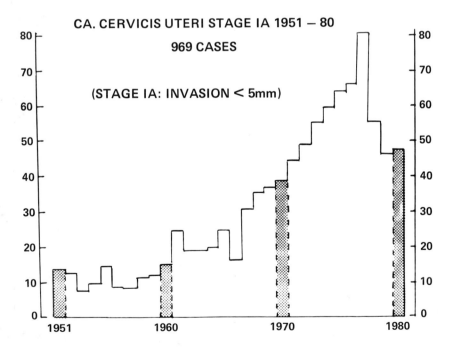

Fig. 7.1. Summary of 969 cases of Ca cervix stage Ia diagnosed during 1951–1980.

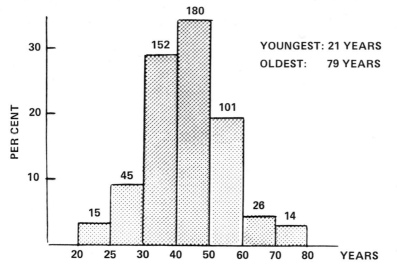

AGE DISTRIBUTION
533 SQUAMOUS CELL MICROCARCINOMAS

YOUNGEST: 21 YEARS
OLDEST: 79 YEARS

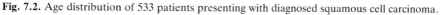

Fig. 7.2. Age distribution of 533 patients presenting with diagnosed squamous cell carcinoma.

Table 7.1. Histological diagnosis in 561 cases of micro-carcinoma of the cervix seen in the period 1971–1980

Squamous cell carcinoma	533
Adenocarcinoma	20
Adenosquamous carcinoma	7
Clear cell carcinoma	1
Total	561

Symptoms

The presenting symptoms are shown in Table 7.2. It has been claimed in the literature that microcarcinoma of the cervix does not produce any symptoms. This is not our experience. In the 1969 study [2] about two-thirds of the patients complained of discharge and spotting, metrorrhagia or contact bleeding. In the present series only one-third had similar suspicious symptoms. The difference between the two series in this respect is most probably related to the fact that today a large percentage of the cases are detected by routine cytology. A total of 205 of the 533 patients (38.5%) with stage Ia squamous cell lesions were found by routine cytology.

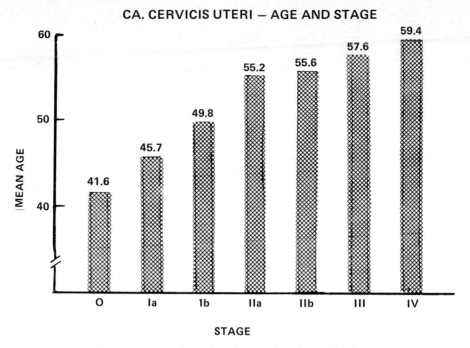

Fig. 7.3. Relation between age at diagnosis and stage of carcinoma, 3474 cases.

Table 7.2. Presenting symptoms in 533 cases of squamous cell carcinoma

	Routine smear	Discharge	Discharge and bleeding	Bleeding	Other
No	205	69	70	125	64
Per cent	38.5	12.9	13.1	23.5	12.0

Cytology

In 375 patients the cytological diagnosis could be compared with the ultimate histological diagnosis (Table 7.3). The number of false negatives is certainly too low, taking into account that 205 cases were detected by routine smear. In approximately one-quarter of the cases the cytopathologist made a diagnosis of CIN III, and in one-third a diagnosis of invasive cancer was predicted. Our cytopathology laboratory has never tried to differentiate between microinvasive and frank invasive carcinoma of the cervix on the basis of the smear pattern. It should be noticed that in stage Ia carcinoma of the cervix, the smear indicated only mild or moderate dysplasia, CIN I–II, in 42.4%.

Table 7.3. Histological diagnosis in 375 patients already assessed by cytology

	Negative	CIN I–II	CIN III	Inv. Ca.
No	11	159	87	118
Per cent	2.9	42.4	23.2	31.5

Colposcopy

Our criteria for making a differential diagnosis between CIN lesions, microinvasive and frank invasive carcinoma have been described in several publications [4,5,6]. In 283 cases in the present series the method of colposcopy, which is primarily dependent upon the vascular pattern and the surface contour of the lesion, was carried out. The findings were classified as indecisive in 13.8% (Table 7.4). The majority of these patients were postmenopausal and the lesion was hidden in the endocervical canal. In 38.5% a CIN grade II–III lesion was suspected, and in 34.6% a correct diagnosis of microcarcinoma was made. Frank invasive carcinoma was predicted in the remaining 13.1% of the cases.

Table 7.4. Diagnosis by colposcopy in 283 patients

	Indecisive	CIN II–III	Micro Ca.	Invasive Ca.
No	39	109	98	37
Per cent	13.8	38.5	34.6	13.1

Treatment

The treatment protocol set up in the early 1970s was as follows: The diagnosis should be made on a cone specimen. A positive diagnosis should be followed by a so-called modified extended hysterectomy with removal of part of the parametria and preservation of the ovaries in the younger age groups. Instead of hysterectomy, postmenopausal patients might receive radium irradiation. If involvement of vessels was found, radical hysterectomy with pelvic lymph node dissection should be the treatment of choice. In older patients the pelvic lymph nodes could also be treated by external radiotherapy without lymphadenectomy.

When reviewing the material many deviations from this treatment protocol were found (Table 7.5). This was to a great extent due to the fact that the majority of the patients were referred from other hospitals after a diagnosis of microcarcinoma had been made, mostly on a cone specimen, but also after simple hysterectomy. The diagnosis was made on a cone specimen in 438 of the 533 cases.

Conisation was considered sufficient treatment in 31 cases, 9 of which represented stump carcinomas where the cervix was extirpated. The remaining 22 had invasion less than 1 mm into the stroma.

Simple hysterectomy performed before referral was also found satisfactory therapy in 25 cases. Extended hysterectomy without conisation was carried out in

Table 7.5. Types of treatment in 533 patients

Treatment	Number
Conisation	31
Simple hysterectomy	25
Extended hysterectomy	51
Conisation +	
simple hysterectomy	62
extended hysterectomy	199
radical hysterectomy and	
lymphadenectomy	42
intracavitary radium	100
external high voltage	
radiation	4
Intracavitary radium	19

51 patients who all had ectocervical lesions easily definable by colposcopy. Primary radium treatment without conisation was given to 19 elderly patients. The diagnosis in these cases was made on colposcopically directed biopsies and endocervical curettage under anaesthesia.

The rest of the patients in the series, 407 cases, were treated according to the protocol described above.

Involved Margins

The surgical specimens were all examined for the presence of carcinomatous tissue in the margins (Table 7.6). It is important to notice that as many as 27.5% of the cone specimens showed involved margins. This is a much higher figure than that found in series of cervical intra-epithelial neoplasia treated by conisation. Even those patients in whom conisation followed a thorough colposcopic examination showed as many as 13.8% with involved margins. This probably reflects the fact that microcarcinoma is a more extensive lesion than cervical intra-epithelial neoplasia and often extends relatively high up into the endocervix.

In the series treated by simple hysterectomy, margins were involved in 4.7%, and in the extended hysterectomy series 1.8%.

Table 7.6. Specimens showing margin involvement

Cone		Hysterectomy		Ext. hysterectomy	
No	%	No	%	No	%
114/415	27.5	3/64	4.7	3/171	1.8

Depth of Infiltration

Depth of infiltration in relation to recurrence and death is shown in Table 7.7. The one patient with a depth of infiltration less than 1 mm who died from cancer was treated for vulvar carcinoma 1 year after conisation for microcarcinoma of the cervix: whether she died from spread from her cervical or vulvar malignancy is uncertain. The other cancer deaths will be described in detail later. There seems to be an increasing risk of recurrence and death with increasing depth of infiltration. Of the ten local recurrences, five had involvement of the margins of the surgical specimen.

Table 7.7. Relation of depth of infiltration to recurrence and death in 533 patients

| | Depth of infiltration | | | |
	< 1 mm	1–2.9 mm	3–5 mm	Total
No	198	168	167	533
Per cent	37.1	31.5	31.3	100
Recurrence	3	4	3	10
Ca. deaths	1 [a]	1	3	5

[a] Ca. vulvae

Wertheim–Meigs Operation

Radical hysterectomy and pelvic lymphadenectomy was performed in 42 patients (Table 7.8). The indications for this procedure in 30 patients was the presence of vessel involvement. In 12 patients a stage Ib lesion was suspected because of the presence of abundant endocervical curettings or of findings at clinical colposcopic examination. Two of these 42 patients had lymph node metastases, one in the parametrium and one in the obturator region. Both had vessel involvement in the cone biopsy specimen.

Complications

Surgical complications are shown in Table 7.9. It is quite obvious that radical hysterectomy with lymphadenectomy carries the highest risk. Of the 42 patients treated in this way, 2 developed urinary fistulas which were successfully treated. Two patients developed lymphocysts which, however, only needed to be treated by aspiration of the cyst fluid. In one case there was a transitory lesion of the femoral nerve, probably caused by the pressure of the self-retaining retractor during operation.

In the series of 250 extended hysterectomies, one intestinal obstruction was treated by re-laparotomy with division of adhesions. Five patients developed

Table 7.8. Indications in 42 patients treated by Wertheim–Meigs operation

No.	Indication
30	Capillary-like space involvement
12	Suspected stage Ib because of findings at clinical and/or colposcopic examination
2	Lymph node metastasis, one in parametrium, one in obturator region

Table 7.9. Surgical complications

42	Wertheim operations	1 Vesico-vaginal fistula
		1 Uretero-vaginal fistula
		2 Lymphocysts
		1 Lymphoedema
		1 Transitory lesion of the femoral nerve
250	Extended hysterectomies	1 Intestinal obstruction
		5 Pelvic infections
		1 Ureteral stenosis
89	Hysterectomies	2 Pelvic infections

pelvic infections, and one patient had a ureteral stenosis with slight reduction in function of one kidney.

Simple hysterectomy in 89 cases was followed in 2 cases by pelvic infection.

Complications after radiotherapy are shown in Table 7.10. After intracavitary radium applications in 119 patients, one patient developed rectal stenosis which had to be treated by temporary colostomy. Another patient developed a bladder ulceration with complicating infections. The ulceration healed spontaneously after 1 year. Four patients received external radiation, and one of these also had a minor rectal stenosis that did not require surgery.

Table 7.10. Complications following radiotherapy

119	Intracavitary radium	1 Rectal stenosis
		1 Bladder ulceration
4	External radiation	2 Rectal stenosis

Follow-up

Table 7.11 shows the treatment methods in the total series both of squamous cell carcinoma and adenocarcinoma, correlated with central (local) recurrences, pelvic wall metastases, distant metastases and deaths. As stated above, of the ten patients with local recurrences in the cervix or vagina, five had involvement of the margins of the surgical specimen. One patient had multiple condylomatous lesions which possibly were not completely removed. Of the lateral (pelvic wall)

Table 7.11. Treatment (all 561 cases) and subsequent histories

| Treatment | Total no. | Recurrence | | | Deaths |
		Central rec.	Lateral rec.	Distant met.	
Conisation	34	3			1
Hysterectomy	94	2			
Ext. hysterectomy	261	4	3	1	4
Wertheim–Meigs	46	1		1	
Radium[a]	126				
Total no.	561	10[b]	3	2	5

a   Ext. radiation: 4
b   Not free margins: 5

recurrences, two out of three had vessel involvement and should have been treated with pelvic lymphadenectomy. The two patients with distant metastases also had vessel involvement. One of these had an adenocarcinoma and massive involvement of vessels and had undergone a Wertheim–Meigs operation, but no metastases were noted in the lymph nodes. Six years after operation massive lung metastases were found and she will certainly die of her disease in the course of a few months.

The case reports for the five patients who have already died from cancer are shown in Table 7.12. It is obvious that vessel involvement cannot be ignored when planning treatment. Furthermore, it is necessary to subject the cone biopsy specimens to rigorous scrutiny in order to detect, or rule out, the presence of tumour cells in capillary-like spaces.

Table 7.12. Case reports on deaths

Patient	Age (years)	History
A.L.	35	Cone 2.5 mm infiltration. Vessel involvement × hysterectomy.
E.J.	45	Lymph nodes not removed. Pelvic wall metastases after 3 and 6 years respectively.
L.S.	35	Cone 4 mm infiltration. Hysterectomy. 6 years later massive spread to the ovaries, upper abdomen, vagina, skin and lungs. Review of cone showed vessel involvement.
J.V.	37	Cone 3–5 mm infiltration. Hysterectomy. 3 years later pelvic and para-aortic metastases. Review of cone did not reveal vessel involvement. Step serial sections not performed.
H.J.	63	Cone < 1 mm infiltration. Free margins. Two years later vulvar carcinoma stage II treated by radical vulvectomy and groin lymphadenectomy. One year later pelvic spread. Cause of death?

Discussion

The three series of stage Ia carcinoma of the cervix presented from our hospital since 1969 confirm numerous reports that this group of lesions has a very good prognosis. Only about 1%–2% of these patients will die from their disease. Of 561 patients treated in the years between 1971 and 1980 only five had died from cancer. We must be aware that some patients will have late recurrences after the usual 5 years of follow-up. The treatment protocol set up in the early 1970s seems in many respects adequate. Especially important is the need to have a cone specimen thoroughly scrutinised for the present or absence of vessel invasion before final therapy is chosen. In the total series of 561 cases, 50 had vessel invasion. Of these, 37 were treated by radical hysterectomy and lymphadenectomy and 4 by external pelvic irradiation. Two patients had lymph node metastases, one in the parametrium and one in the obturator region. However, none of these 41 patients has to date developed pelvic recurrences or distant metastases.

In nine cases, for a reason at present obscure, the lymph nodes were not treated, in spite of clear-cut signs of vessel invasion. Of these nine patients, three have developed metastases and died.

As for the rest of the series—a total of 501 patients—it may be seriously questioned whether our treatment policy has been too radical. It seems obvious from our experience that infiltration less that 1 mm does not call for further therapy (Table 7.13). Moreover, lesions invading less that 3 mm may most probably be safely treated by conisation alone provided there are ample free margins and no signs of vessel invasion. Simple hysterectomy should possibly be recommended for lesions invading between 3 and 5 mm with free margins. If the margins are involved, however, one can never be certain that there is no deeper lesion left behind, and extended hysterectomy is the safest procedure.

A last modification would be that when conisation has removed the whole lesion, but vessel invasion is found, it is probably not necessary to perform radical hysterectomy. Simple hysterectomy with lymph node dissection, or even lymphadenectomy only, should be adequate treatment. In this way some of the more serious complications connected with Wertheim hysterectomy may be avoided.

Table 7.13. Treatment of choice in various circumstances: stage Ia Ca cervix diagnosed by conisation

Proposed treatment	Free margins invasion		Not free margins	Vessel invasion
	Minimal	1–5 mm		
No further therapy	X	(X)		
Hysterectomy		X		
Extended hysterectomy			X	
Hysterectomy and lymphadenectomy				X
Radium		(X)		
Ext. irradiation				(X)

Definitional Problems

There is still no international agreement in existence on the definition of microinvasive carcinoma of the cervix, or carcinoma of the cervix stage Ia. A study group of the Royal College of Obstetricians and Gynaecologists in 1981 proposed the following definition [7]:

Stage Ia (microinvasive carcinoma) is a histological diagnosis.
Two groups should be recognised:

1. *Early (minimal) stromal invasion*
   Buds are found in continuity with an in situ lesion, or separated cells may be found not more than 1 mm from the nearest surface or crypt membrane.
2. *Measurable lesions*
   These should be measured in two dimensions: The depth should be measured from the base of the epithelium from which it develops and should not exceed 5 mm. The diameter in the slide which shows the largest extent should not exceed 10 mm.

It was recommended by the Ninth Study Group of the Royal College that this definition should be used in the years to come to enable the collection of sufficient and comparable material.

If vessel invasion is found, it should not influence the staging, but it should be reported when the series is published. Preferably also, so-called confluency of tumour cells should be included in the reporting.

References

1. Mestwerdt G (1951) Elektive Therapie des Mikrokarzinoms am Collum Uteri? Zentralbl Gynakol 73:558–567
2. Kolstad P (1969) Carcinoma of the cervix stage Ia. Am J Obstet Gynecol 104:1015–1022
3. Iversen T, Abeler V, Kjørstad KE (1979) Factors influencing the treatment of patients with stage Ia carcinoma of the cervix. Br J Obstet Gynaecol 86:593–597
4. Johannisson E, Kolstad P, Søderberg G (1966) Cytologic, vascular and histologic patterns of dysplasia, carcinoma in situ and early invasive carcinoma of the cervix. Acta Radiol [Suppl] 258
5. Kolstad P (1976) Colposcopic diagnosis of cervical neoplasia. In: Jordan JA, Singer A (eds) The cervix. Saunders, London
6. Kolstad P, Stafl A (1982) Atlas of colposcopy. 3rd edn. Universitetsforlaget, Oslo
7. Jordan JA, Sharp F, Singer A (eds) (1981) Pre-clinical neoplasia of the cervix. Proceedings of the Ninth Study Group of the Royal College of Obstetricians and Gynaecologists, p 302

8 · Radical Hysterectomy and Pelvic Lymphadenectomy, 1974–1982

J.L. Powell, S.R. Mogelnicki, M.O. Burrell, E.W. Franklin and D.A. Chambers

Introduction

The first part of this paper is concerned with the review of a 9-year experience of radical hysterectomy and pelvic lymphadenectomy, and the second part is a discussion of the marked improvements in intra-operative care that have occurred as a result of the institution of controlled hypotension.

Of the 250 patients operated on between 1974 and 1982, 197 were white, 54 black, 3 Asian and 1 American Indian. They ranged in age from 15 to 78 with a mean of 41 years. The age distribution of the patients is shown in Table 8.1, with 74.9% of the patients under the age of 50. This would indicate that the majority of patients had a long life expectancy if they could be cured of their disease.

Table 8.1. Age distribution of 255 patients

Age group	No. of patients	%
15–19	3	1.2
20–29	38	14.9
30–39	94	36.9
40–49	56	21.9
50–59	38	14.9
60–69	22	8.6
70–78	4	1.6

Type and Location of Cancers

All but 4 patients had primary cervical carcinoma. Two patients were being treated for stage II occult adenocarcinoma of the endometrium and 2 diethylstilboestrol-exposed progeny were treated for clear cell adenocarcinoma of the vagina (ages 19 and 23). Of the 251 primary cervical carcinomas, 80.9% were squamous cell, 13.9% were adenocarcinoma and 4.4% were mixed adeno-squamous carcinoma. Of the 251 cervical carcinomas, 5 were stage Ia done during the earlier years of this study. Our present practice in stage Ia disease is to perform radical hysterectomy only if lymphatic or vascular invasion or confluent areas of microinvasive tumour are present. A total of 233 were stage Ib and 13 were stage IIa. There were 3 patients with a cervical stump and 7 patients were pregnant at the time of their surgery. Two operations were performed at 10 weeks' gestation, one operation was done at $29\frac{1}{2}$ weeks' gestation after steroid induction of fetal lung maturity and 4 were performed in conjunction with classical caesarean section at term. The average hospital stay was 13.1 days.

Postoperative Complications

The operative mortality was 0.78%. One patient had a cardiac arrest on the 5th postoperative day, and one patient had a massive pulmonary embolus on the 14th postoperative day. Four other patients with pulmonary emboli were treated with full anticoagulation and recovered. Mini-doses of heparin had been given as a routine prophylactic measure to all patients. Table 8.2 shows the operative

Table 8.2. Operative mortality rates with radical hysterectomy

Author [Ref.]	Year	No. of patients	No. of operative deaths	Mortality rate (%)
Liu and Meigs [1]	1955	473	8	1.69
Brunschwig [2]	1960	149	1	0.67
Masterson [3]	1967	180	2	1.11
Park [4]	1973	150	1	0.66
Morley [5]	1976	208	3	1.44
Hoskins [6]	1976	224	2	0.89
Mikuta [7]	1977	243	2	0.82
Sall [8]	1979	349	0	0
Webb [9]	1979	610	2	0.33
Underwood [10]	1979	178	0	0
Langley [11]	1980	284	0	0
Bonar [12]	1980	96	1	1.04
Benedet [13]	1980	241	1	0.41
Lerner [14]	1980	108	1	0.93
Mann [15]	1981	207	1	0.48
Powell (this study)	1983	255	2	0.78

mortality rates in all reported series in the past 28 years. Our experience compares favourably with that reported by others.

The types of postoperative complications are shown in Table 8.3. The usual postoperative problems associated with abdominal and pelvic surgery, such as transient ileus, atelectasis, urinary tract infection, phlebitis, and wound infection were encountered. All responded to the usual postoperative management methods. Postoperative bowel obstruction occurred in three patients, all of whom required operative intervention. Two merely needed lysis of adhesions, while one had resection of an infarcted segment of ileum and end-to-end anastomosis. Seven patients had prolonged bladder dysfunction and three of these had to be taught self-catheterisation. Of our patients 51% were voiding spontaneously with minimal residual urine volumes within 2 weeks of surgery, and the majority of others within a month.

There were six patients with urinary tract fistulae. Each of these patients had several factors in common which pre-disposed them to poor healing and the development of this complication, including previous pelvic surgery, diabetes mellitus, obesity, hypertension and superimposed pelvic infection. The two ureteric fistulae both healed spontaneously over indwelling ureteric stents. One vesico-vaginal fistula closed spontaneously after treatment with an indwelling Foley catheter and two of the vesico-vaginal fistulae were subsequently successfully repaired surgically. The other patient with a vesico-vaginal fistula

Table 8.3. Postoperative complications

Type	No. of patients	%
Intestinal		
Ileus	10	3.9
Obstruction	3	1.2
Urinary		
Infection	10	3.9
Vesical fistula	4	1.6
Ureteral fistula	2	0.8
Prolonged bladder atony	7	2.7
Wound		
Infection	5	2.0
Evisceration	0	0
Pulmonary		
Atelectasis	7	2.7
Pneumonia	1	0.4
Embolism	5	2.0
Pelvic		
Abscess	5	2.0
Cellulitis	8	3.1
Haematoma	5	2.0
Lymphocyst	2	0.8
Medical		
Thrombophlebitis	7	2.7
Lymphoedema	2	0.8
Congestive heart failure	1	0.4
Sepsis	2	0.8
Postoperative Haemorrhage		
Vaginal	1	0.4
Intra- or retro-peritoneal	4	1.6

developed bilateral ureteric obstruction due to retroperitoneal fibrosis and was managed by urinary diversion. There were no recto-vaginal fistulae.

The recently published fistula rates in most large centres in which radical pelvic surgery is common practice are shown in Table 8.4. Much higher fistula rates occurred in the earlier years of other series before the use of retroperitoneal suction drainage which, combined with prophylactic antibiotics, has significantly reduced the incidence of pelvic infection and in so doing has also significantly decreased the fistula rate.

Table 8.4. Urinary fistula rate as a complication of radical hysterectomy

Author [Ref.]	Years of study	No. of cases	No. of fistulae	Percentage of fistulae
Masterson [3]	1950–1964	180	9	5.00
Morley [5]	1945–1975	208	11	5.29
Hoskins [6]	1965–1974	224	6	2.68
Macasaet [16]	1964–1969	72	7	9.72
Macasaet [16]	1969–1973	70	1	1.43
Mikuta [7]	1955–1976	243	31	12.76
Sall [8]	1963–1977	349	10	2.86
Webb [9]	1956–1975	610	29	4.75
Underwood [10]	1956–1978	178	14	7.86
Langley [11]	1950–1975	284	20	7.04
Bonar [12]	1947–1977	96	5	5.21
Benedet [13]	1949–1978	247	22	8.91
Lerner [14]	1963–1977	108	1	0.93
Mann [15]	1969–1979	207	2	0.97
Powell (this study)	1974–1982	255	6	2.35

Recurrence

Microscopic metastatic carcinoma to the regional lymph nodes was discovered in 30 patients for an incidence of 11.8%. One of the two patients with stage II endometrial carcinoma had microscopic lymph node metastases. Among the patients with cervical cancer, none of the patients with stage Ia disease and 28 of 233 patients with stage Ib (12%) had lymph node metastases. In our series, the cell type of the tumour did not influence the incidence of nodal metastases, but increasing tumour size and degree of de-differentiation correlated strongly with an increasing incidence of lymph node involvement (see Table 8.5).

At present 24 of the 30 patients with positive nodes are known to be alive with no evidence of disease (80%), and 6 have died due to their malignancy. Nine patients had focal metastasis to a single node and one patient had bilateral parametrial nodes involved focally in the subcapsular sinus. All ten of these patients were treated with surgery only, and all ten are living and free of disease. Of the patients with either extensive involvement of one node or multiple nodal metastases, 20 received postoperative external pelvic radiation therapy [5000 cGy (rad)], of whom 14 are now alive (70%).

Table 8.5. Pelvic node metastases according to tumour grade

Histologic grade	Series of 255		With positive nodes	
	No.	%	No.	%
1	77	30.2	2	6.7
2	108	42.4	12	40.0
3	70	27.4	16	53.3

Postoperative total pelvic irradiation was utilised in ten patients with micro-scopically positive or close surgical margins; eight are living and well, one died of her malignancy, and one was lost to follow-up.

Recurrent tumour has appeared in 16 of the 255 patients (6.3%). Of these 16, 14 have died due to cancer.

The status of all 255 patients treated is illustrated in Table 8.6. There were two patients lost to follow-up, two operative mortalities, and two deaths due to intercurrent disease. At the last appraisal, 235 (92%) of the women were living and well and 14 (5.5%) had died of cancer. Among those patients eligible for 5-year analysis, the survival rate is 90.3% (93 of 103 patients).

Table 8.6. Causes of death, cases lost to follow-up and survival by site and stage

Site and stage	No. of cases	Dead				Cases lost to follow-up	Survivors	
		Total	Operative mortality	Recurrence	Intercurrent disease		No.	%
Cervix								
Ia	5	0	0	0	0	0	5	100
Ib	233	14	0	13	1	2	217	93
IIa	13	3	2	0	1	0	10	77
Endometrium								
II	2	1	0	1	0	0	1	50
Vagina								
I	2	0	0		0	0	2	100
Total	255	18	2	14	2	2	235	92

New Hypotensive Anaesthetic Technique

The average operating time was 4 h and 15 min and the average blood loss was 943 ml. At the first review of our data in 1980 [17] the blood loss averaged 1264 ml and 84% of patients were being transfused. Given the risks associated with blood transfusions (see Table 8.7), this rate seemed too high. A new technique was devised by two of the authors (J.L.P. and S.R.M.) which we have continued to use because of the dramatic results achieved.

During the past two years of this study we have, in 86 cases, employed a deliberate controlled hypotensive anaesthetic technique utilising intravenous nitroglycerine (a vasodilator) in order to reduce mean arterial blood pressure and

Table 8.7. Transfusion problems

O$_2$–hgb dissociation
Acid-base balance
Temperature
Coagulation
Hyperkalaemia
Citrate toxification
Hepatitis
Shock lung
AIDS[a]

[a]   Acquired immune deficiency syndrome

thus (a) reduce operative blood loss, (b) decrease the number of blood transfusions needed, (c) shorten operating time and improve surgical dissection by producing a relatively dry operative field. Only the reports of Linacre [18] of Sussex in 1961 and Ditzler and Eckenhoff [19] of Pennsylvania in 1956 utilising ganglion blockers and regional anaesthesia provide any published experience regarding the use of this anaesthetic technique for gynaecological surgery.

The practical advantages of deliberate hypotension, although at times debatable and sometimes misunderstood, become obvious when attempting an extensive and potentially haemorrhagic surgical dissection. The incentive to reduce the amount of blood loss is increased when patients have rare blood types, are difficult to crossmatch, or refuse blood transfusions for religious or other reasons (hepatitis, AIDS).

A sterile aqueous solution of nitroglycerine (0.2 mg per ml of 5% dextrose in water) was prepared by the hospital pharmacy and infused at a rate of 0.5–5 µg/kg per minute. Nitroglycerine was titrated to keep a mean blood pressure at 60 mmHg (8 kPa). The infusion was discontinued and blood pressure returned to normal before closing the pelvic peritoneum in order to ensure adequate haemostasis. All patients were hydrated with crystalloid and plasma volume expanders to maintain a central venous pressure (CVP) of 7 cm. All patients were monitored with V5 precordial electrocardiogram, direct intra-arterial pressures, CVP, urine output, temperature, arterial blood gases, electrolytes, and serial haematocrit and haemoglobin determinations.

Nitroglycerine is extremely evanescent in its action. Hypotension is produced within 2–3 min and recovery occurs in 6–9 min. Excessive cooling of the patient related to the vasodilated state and the air-conditioned environment of the operating room was prevented by warming intravenous fluids and inspired gases, and by the use of a thermal blanket.

We chose nitroglycerine over sodium nitroprusside (another vasodilator) because nitroglycerine has negligible toxicity, whereas sodium nitroprusside is metabolised to cyanide and thiocyanate with significant toxic potential if doses above 8–10 µg/kg per minute are exceeded.

Results

The details, efficiency and safety of this technique, based on statistical analysis of an initial pilot study of 26 patients, was published in September 1983 [20] (see

Table 8.8. Comparison of blood loss, transfusion rate, operating time, hospital stay (mean ± SE)

	1980 control group	Hypotensive group, 1981	P value
Mean blood loss (ml)	1133 ± 247	331 ± 65	<0.001[a]
Transfusion rate (%)	81	11.5	<0.001[b]
Operating time (h)	4.33 ± 0.33	3.05 ± 0.60	<0.001[a]
Hospital stay (d)	13.5 ± 2.9	11.6 ± 2.3	<0.10[a]

[a]   Student t-test
[b]   Chi-squared test

Table 8.8). The objectives were all met in this pilot study with P values of <0.001. The main criticism of this study was the use of historical controls from the immediately preceding year. However, the results were so dramatic that it seemed unethical to randomise the patients, especially as there had been no change in the surgical and anaesthetic teams, or in the guidelines for giving blood.

With expansion of the study group to 86 cases, in 1981 and 1982, we have reduced the estimated operative blood loss to an average of 508 ml and results continue to improve with time and experience (so far this year average blood loss has been 300 ml). The percentage of patients requiring transfusions has been reduced from 84% to 30%. The mean operating time has been 3 h and 27 min—a reduction of 25% when compared with those who did not undergo this deliberate hypotensive technique. A comparison of admission and discharge haematocrits between the control and study groups showed no significant difference (admission haematocrit 41.0% vs. 39.9%; discharge haematocrit 35.5% vs 33.5).

There were no operative deaths or fistulae in this recent study group, and no patient experienced any complication related to alteration of cardiovascular haemodynamics. There have been no cerebral, cardiac, renal, pulmonary, or hepatic complications. That is to say, there has been no evidence of altered mental function, psychological alterations, or altered functions of major organs related to decreased regional blood flow detected in follow-up interviews, physical examination, electro-cardiograms or biochemical profiles.

Discussion

The indications for controlled hypotension are still controversial and somewhat dependent upon local practice, blood availability, and the risk of hepatitis associated with available blood. The decision to employ deliberate hypotension must be a joint understanding between surgeon and anaesthetist. The suggestion for its use should originate in advance of surgery, and either party should be able to veto the plan if the patient is considered a poor risk, if the benefits to be gained are not sufficient to warrant its use, or if the anaesthetist's experience with the technique is inadequate. The request for, and the decision to use, a hypotensive technique should rarely be instituted after surgery has begun.

The production of hypotension by any means is considered contra-indicated in patients with inadequate cerebral circulation. In general, cerebrovascular disease, myocardial ischaemia, hypertension, peripheral vascular disease, chronic obstructive pulmonary disease, severe renal or hepatic disease and hypovolaemia are contra-indications to deliberate hypotension. An anaesthetist's inexperience with the technique is perhaps the most important contra-indication to its use.

Our data clearly demonstrate that deliberate hypotension employing nitro-glycerine for radical hysterectomies is a safe, effective and cost-saving technique. Using this technique, we have significantly reduced operating time, blood loss and need for transfusion.

Given the favourable results for survival, freedom from recurrence, minimal late sequelae, and low rates of serious surgical complications—added to the advantages of ovarian conservation and preservation of a functional vagina, in contrast to the results of radiation therapy—radical hysterectomy with pelvic lymphadenectomy is an excellent form of therapy for selected patients with early invasive cervical cancer.

References

1. Liu W, Meigs JV (1955) Radical hysterectomy and pelvic lymphadenectomy. Am J Obstet Gynecol 69:1–32
2. Brunschwig A (1960) Surgical treatment of Stage I cancer of the cervix. Cancer 13:34–36
3. Masterson JG (1967) The role of surgery in the treatment of early carcinoma of the cervix. Clin Obstet Gynecol 10:922–938
4. Park RC, Patow WE, Rogers RR, Zimmerman EA (1973) Treatment of Stage I carcinoma of the cervix. Obstet Gynecol 41:117–122
5. Morley GW, Seski JC (1976) Radical pelvic surgery versus radiation therapy for Stage I carcinoma of the cervix (exclusive of microinvasion). Am J Obstet Gynecol 126:785–798
6. Hoskins WJ, Ford JH, Lutz MH, Averette HE (1976) Radical hysterectomy and pelvic lymphadenectomy for the management of early invasive cancer of the cervix. Gynecol Oncol 4:278–290
7. Mikuta JJ, Giuntoli RL, Rubin EL, Mangan CE (1977) The 'problem' radical hysterectomy. Am J Obstet Gynecol 128:119–127
8. Sall S, Pineda AA, Calanog A, Heller P, Greenberg H (1979) Surgical treatment of Stages Ib and IIa invasive carcinoma of the cervix by radical abdominal hysterectomy. Am J Obstet Gynecol 135:442–446
9. Webb MJ, Symmonds RE (1979) Wertheim hysterectomy: A reappraisal. Obstet Gynecol 54:140–145
10. Underwood PB Jr, Wilson WC, Kreutner A, Miller MC, Murphy E (1979) Radical hysterectomy: A critical review of twenty-two years' experience. Am J Obstet Gynecol 134:889–898
11. Langley II, Moore DW, Tarnasky JW, Roberts PHR (1980) Radical hysterectomy and pelvic lymph node dissection. Gynecol Oncol 9:37–42
12. Bonar LD (1980) Results of radical surgical procedures after radiation for treatment of invasive carcinoma of the uterine cervix in a private practice. Am J Obstet Gynecol 136:1006–1008
13. Benedet JL, Turko M, Boyes DA, Nickerson KG, Bienkowska BT (1980) Radical hysterectomy in the treatment of cervical cancer. Am J Obstet Gynecol 137:254–262
14. Lerner HM, Jones HW, Hill EC (1980) Radical surgery for the treatment of early invasive cervical carcinoma (stage Ib): Review of 15 years' experience. Obstet Gynecol 56:413–416
15. Mann WJ, Orr JW Jr, Shingleton HM et al. (1981) Perioperative influences on infectious morbidity in radical hysterectomy. Gynecol Oncol 11:207–212
16. Macasaet MA, Lu T, Nelson JH Jr (1976) Ureterovaginal fistula as a complication of radical pelvic surgery. Am J. Obstet Gynecol 124:757–760
17. Powell JL, Burrell MO, Franklin EW (1981) Radical hysterectomy and pelvic lymphadenectomy. Gynecol Oncol 12:23–32
18. Linacre JL (1961) Induced hypotension in gynaecological surgery. Br J Anaesth 33:45–50

19. Ditzler JW, Eckenhoff JE (1956) A comparison of blood loss and operative time in certain surgical procedures completed with and without controlled hypotension. Ann Surg 143:289–293
20. Powell JL, Mogelnicki SR, Franklin EW, Chambers DA, Burrell MO (1983) A deliberate hypotensive technique for decreasing blood loss during radical hysterectomy and pelvic lymphadenectomy. Am J Obstet Gynecol 147:196–202

9 · Intra-operative Radiation Therapy for Cervical Carcinoma*

E.S. Petrilli, G. Delgado and A.L. Goldson

Introduction

Conventional radiation therapy fails to control advanced cervical cancer in many patients despite the modern technical advances of megavoltage delivery systems. Patients with extensive regional tumour or metastatic carcinoma to para-aortic lymph nodes continue to be at high risk of treatment failure and death from disease. Para-aortic treatment has not improved survival, although the high morbidity related to transperitoneal lymphadenectomy and extended field therapy has been markedly decreased by retroperitoneal staging procedures and reduced radiation doses [1]. In an attempt to improve the outcome for patients with advanced tumours, a variety of investigational methods, including particle beam therapy, hyperthermia, radiation sensitisers, and intra-operative radiation therapy, are currently under study.

Although interest in intra-operative therapy has existed throughout much of this century, the modern era of investigation began in Japan twenty years ago when the first betatron was placed in an operating room [2]. The potential advantage of intra-operative therapy is its capacity to overcome tumour dose limitations imposed by the tolerance of surrounding normal tissues. When a tumour site is exposed at operation, a single high-energy dose is delivered directly to that area while intestinal and urinary tract tissues are excluded from the treatment field. For cervical cancer, conventional radiotherapy has been administered after postoperative recovery from intra-operative therapy. This results in a higher effective tumour dose than can be achieved by standard therapy alone.

* Reprinted with permission of the American College of Obstetricians and Gynecologists and the publishers of the journal *Obstetrics and Gynecology* (1984) 63:246–252.

Despite the experience in the literature of over 1000 patients with various tumours who have been treated by intra-operative therapy, many basic questions remain unanswered in regard to treatment indications, effectiveness, optimal doses and complications [3–6]. The relationship of intra-operative therapy to cancer surgery and external beam therapy in various sequences and combinations also requires further investigation. This report describes the results of intra-operative therapy for patients with advanced cervical cancer who were considered to have high risk for treatment failure by conventional treatment methods.

Methods

From 1978 to 1983, 19 patients between 27 and 72 years of age (average 52 years) with stage II, III, IV or recurrent/persistent carcinoma of the cervix were treated with intra-operative radiotherapy at Georgetown University and Howard University Hospitals. Sixteen patients had squamous carcinoma and three had adenocarcinoma. Sixteen patients had received no prior therapy for their disease. Three others who had recurrent or persistent cancer limited to the pelvis after conventional radiation therapy were not suitable for pelvic exenteration. Each patient had a pretreatment history and physical examination, chest X-ray, intravenous pyelogram, cystoscopy, barium enema, proctoscopy and lymphangiogram or computed tomography scan. Some patients had percutaneous fine-needle aspiration biopsy of lymph nodes that were abnormal by radiographic evaluation.

Patients were treated at the Howard University intra-operative radiation facility where a Varian Clinac 18 MeV linear accelerator is located in a modified operating room in the radiation medicine department (Fig. 9.1). The electron beam is used because it delivers a relatively superficial and homogeneous dose that limits treatment of normal structures deep to the target site. The desired depth of treatment is proportional to the energy of the beam that is selected, i.e. 6, 9, 12 or 18 MeV [7]. A Lucite applicator is placed into the opened abdomen to delineate the treatment field and then attached to an anodised aluminium anti-crush device joined to the collimator of the linear accelerator.

At laparotomy, bilateral para-aortic lymphadenectomy was performed. If lymph nodes were unresectable, biopsies were obtained to confirm the presence of cancer. The small bowel and ureters were retracted from the treatment field and a Lucite applicator was positioned in the abdomen over the para-aortic area and packed in place (Fig. 9.2). After positioning beneath the linear accelerator, the operating table was elevated to join the Lucite applicator and the aluminium attachment of the collimator (Fig. 9.3). Treatment was administered while the patient was alone in the operating room with the anaesthetist nearby monitoring a continuous video display of vital functions.

After para-aortic therapy was completed, the pelvis and the retroperitoneal spaces were explored. Pelvic lymph nodes were resected and when this was not possible biopsies were obtained. The ureters, sigmoid colon and bladder were retracted medially, and a Lucite applicator was inserted into the pelvis to define the treatment field, which included the pelvic sidewall and the lymph nodes from the aortic bifurcation to the distal external iliac artery. Overlap with the para-

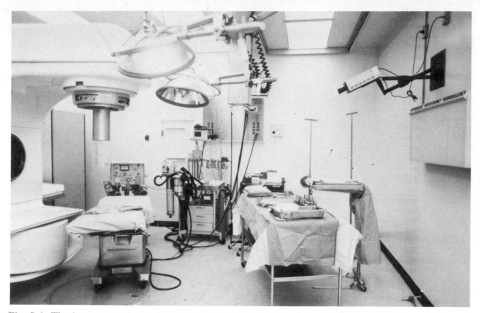

Fig. 9.1. The intra-operative radiation facility in the Department of Radiation Medicine at Howard University has a Clinac 18 MeV linear accelerator located in a modified operating room with radiation shielding.

aortic field was avoided. A summary of the intra-operative treatment protocol is presented in Table 9.1. Patients with negative lymph nodes received 1500 cGy (rad) to the para-aortic area and those with microscopic metastases received 2000 cGy. Patients with unresectable positive nodes received 2500 cGy of intra-operative therapy and an additional 2500 cGy at a later date by external beam extended field therapy. For microscopic metastases to pelvic lymph nodes, 1500 cGy were delivered and unresectable pelvic nodes were treated with 2500 cGy. Patients with invisible parametrial disease received an additional 2500 cGy to that area.

After a 10–14 day period of postoperative recovery, conventional radiotherapy was started for patients undergoing primary therapy. The treatment plan included 4500–5000 cGy by external beam to the whole pelvis and extended field therapy of 2500 cGy to T-12 for patients who had unresectable disease in para-aortic lymph nodes. Two weeks after completion of external beam therapy, an intracavitary system was inserted for 48 h and a second application followed 2 weeks later.

Results

Of 16 patients with previously untreated cancer, 11 had positive para-aortic nodes and 5 were negative. All of these patients received para-aortic therapy and 8 also had treatment to the pelvic lymph nodes and, when, indicated, to the parametria

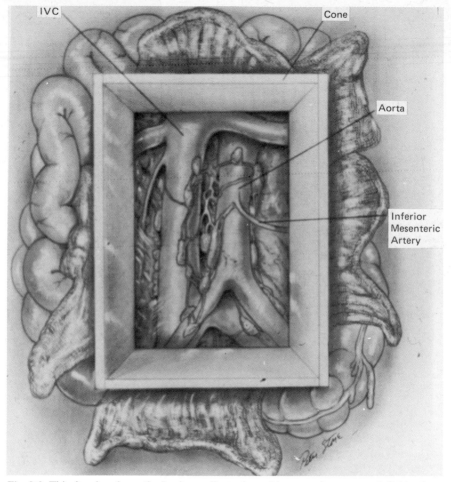

Fig. 9.2. This drawing shows the Lucite applicator in position over the para-aortic field to be treated.

as well[1]. All patients in this group later received external beam therapy. Twelve patients had two intracavitary applications and two patients had only one insertion each. Some patients did not complete planned therapy for various reasons that included medical complications, withdrawal from treatment, and death from rapid disease progression. Of ten patients, three had recurrent or persistent pelvic cancer and negative para-aortic lymph nodes. They received only intra-operative therapy to the parametrial and pelvic sidewall sites of recurrence (Table 9.2).

The outcome of the 11 patients with positive para-aortic nodes is summarised in Table 9.3. Eight patients who died of disease had an average survival of 7 months. One patient is alive with disease. Two patients died of treatment complications. One had no clinical evidence of disease, and the other had a small volume of persistent disease confirmed at operation. Of five patients with negative para-

---

[1] When the study was begun only the para-aortic area was treated. This was later changed to include the pelvic lymph nodes and, when tumour was present, the parametria as well.

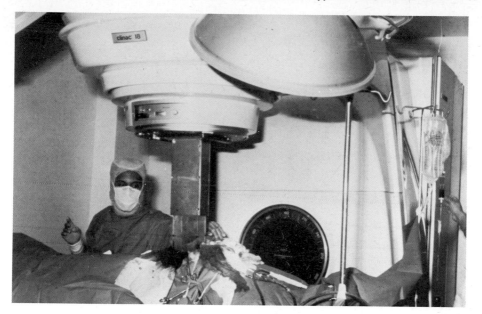

Fig. 9.3. The Lucite field applicator has been placed in the abdominal cavity and joined to the collimator of the linear accelerator.

Table 9.1. Treatment plan for radiation therapy

	Dose (cGy)	Energy (MeV)
Intraoperative radiation		
Para-aortic area[a]		
Negative nodes	−1500	9–12
Positive Nodes		
A. Microscopic metastasis (surgically removed)	2000	9–12
B. Grossly positive (biopsy only)	2500	
Pelvic area: lymph nodes		
A. Microscopic metastasis	1500	9–12
B. Grossly positive nodes	2500	12
Parametria	2500	
External radiation		
Para-aortic nodes (unresectable)	2500	12
Pelvis	4500–5000	
Intracavitary applications		
Pelvis	2 applications (48 h each)	

[a]   Administered to all patients having primary treatment.

Table 9.2. Radiation therapy and lymph node status

	Patients		
	Para-aortic nodes		
Radiation therapy	Pos.[b]	Neg.[c]	Total
All modalities	11	8	19
Intraoperative radiation			
Para-aortic nodes	11	5	16
Pelvic nodes/parametria	6	2	8
Pelvic side wall[a]	0	3	3
External radiation			
Prior to intra-operative radiation	0	3	3
Following intra-operative radiation	10	6	16
Intracavitary application			
Single	2	0	2
Double	5	7	12

[a] These patients received pelvic intra-operative therapy alone for recurrent/persistent cervical cancer after conventional radiation therapy failed to cure their disease.
[b] Pos. = metastases present
[c] Neg. = metastases absent

aortic nodes, two are disease free, one is alive with disease, one died of intercurrent disease and one died of treatment complications (Table 9.4). Three patients had intra-operative therapy after conventional radiotherapy failed to cure their cancer, and all had disease involving the pelvic sidewall that was not surgically resectable. Two of these patients subsequently died of disease at 3 and 36 months after intra-operative therapy. One patient remains disease free 2 years after treatment.

Treatment complications are listed in Table 9.5. Two patients died of arterial haemorrhage related to pelvic necrosis and disruption of the hypogastric artery. One of these patients had vaginal vault necrosis and haemorrhage months after

Table 9.3. Primary treatment. Outcome in 11 patients with positive para-aortic lymph nodes. Stage II, 2 patients; stage III, 7 patients; stage IV, 2 patients

Outcome	
Dead of disease	8
Dead of treatment complications	2[a]
Alive with disease	1
Disease location	
Pelvis	4
Pelvis + distant	5
Survival after therapy (months)	
Average	7
Range	2–17

[a] Despite surgical intervention, one patient died of hypogastric arterial haemorrhage related to pelvic necrosis. Tumour was present on a segment of sigmoid colon resected at the time of operation. No cancer was found at the site of arterial disruption. The other patient was free of tumour at surgical exploration performed to determine if cancer was the cause of pelvic pain and neurological deficit of the lumbar plexus. The patient died 8 months later of sepsis and pelvic abscess and was still clinically free of tumour although autopsy was not performed.

Table 9.4. Primary treatment. Outcome in 5 patients with negative para-aortic nodes. Stage II, 3 patients; stage III, 2 patients

Outcome	
Dead of disease	0
Dead of treatment complications	1[a]
Dead of intercurrent disease	1
Alive with disease	1
No evidence of disease	2
Survival after therapy (months)	
Average	20
Range	4–30

[a] This patient died of hypogastric arterial haemorrhage 6 months after urinary diversion for ureteric obstruction due to pelvic fibrosis. No cancer was found at autopsy.

Table 9.5. Complications related to operation and radiation therapy

Complications	No. of cases
Arterial haemorrhage	2[a]
Radiation neuritis	2
Pelvic abscess	1[a]
Ureteric obstruction	1
Vena cava laceration	2
Leg oedema	3
Prolonged ileus	2

[a] Three patients had fatal treatment complications. One was free of disease, one had a small volume of residual disease, and one was clinically free of disease without post-mortem confirmation.

completion of intra-operative radiation therapy. When arterial embolisation failed to control the bleeding, laparotomy was performed. Extensive pelvic necrosis was present and the completely disrupted right hypogastric artery was ligated near the defect close to the common iliac artery. Necrosis of the sigmoid colon required resection and colostomy, and tumour was found in the specimen on pathological examination. The patient later experienced a fatal recurrent haemorrhage. The second patient required ileoneocystotomy 8 months after intra-operative therapy for left ureteric obstruction caused by extensive pelvic fibrosis. Three months later the patient presented with vaginal haemorrhage that was incompletely controlled by arterial embolisation and bleeding persisted. She refused further treatment and expired. Autopsy revealed rupture of the left hypogastric artery 5 mm below the common iliac bifurcation in an area adjacent to a necrotic lymph node. No tumour was present.

Two instances of neurological injury occurred. One patient manifested a unilateral femoral nerve deficit. The other had severe pelvic pain and muscle weakness of the legs. Neurological evaluation resulted in a differential diagnosis of radiation neuritis versus tumour involvement of the lumbar plexus. At operation no tumour was found although extensive pelvic fibrosis was present. The left ureter was damaged during the difficult dissection and required re-anastomosis. Persistent postoperative leakage occurred from a drain placed near the ureteric repair, even though a nephrostomy had been previously performed for obstructive uropathy. Eight months later the patient died of sepsis related to a left pelvic abscess. She was still clinically free of cancer. A post-mortem examination was not obtained.

The two vena cava injuries and three instances of prolonged ileus were surgical complications unrelated to intra-operative radiation per se.

Discussion

Of the 16 patients who had primary treatment, only two are alive and free of disease and both had negative para-aortic lymph nodes. Although these results do not demonstrate a survival advantage over conventional therapy alone, the methods used demonstrated the capacity to reduce and in some cases completely eradicate large volumes of tumour. One of the three patients with recurrent cancer is alive and free of disease 2 years after treatment. Patients with recurrent or persistent regional disease not suitable for pelvic exenteration may be good candidates for intra-operative therapy because of the limited treatment alternatives available in this situation. With regard to future investigation, intra-operative therapy used in conjunction with cisplatinum may be of interest in such cases. Workers at the National Cancer Institute are investigating a combined modality approach for synergistic effects using misonidazole as a radiation sensitiser and intra-operative radiotherapy [8]

Although intra-operative radiation used in conjunction with conventional therapy has demonstrated a capacity to reduce large tumour volumes in this study, it did not appreciably alter the pattern of failure because all patients who died of disease had persistent regional cancer with or without distant metastases.

Two patients died from hypogastric arterial disruption and haemorrhage related to vascular necrosis as a result of treatment. One was free of cancer and the other had small residual disease. One of these patients also had a preceding complication with ureteric obstruction due to pelvic fibrosis that required operative correction. A third patient was clinically free of disease when she died of pelvic abscess and sepsis. This patient also suffered radiation neuritis of the lumbar plexus as a result of treatment.

Only recently have studies been done to define the tolerance of normal tissues to intra-operative therapy. Although the biological effects of single high-dose treatment are not well understood, they appear to exceed those of similar doses delivered by standard fractionation. In dogs, histological disruption of the intima and fibrosis of the media of the aorta occur with single intra-operative doses of 3000 cGy or more [7]. Atherosclerotic blood vessels in older patients with cervical cancer are likely to be more sensitive to injury than normal tissues. The patients who had vascular and neurological complications in this report received intra-operative doses of 1500–2500 cGy to these structures and an additional dose of approximately 6000 cGy derived from subsequent external beam and intracavitary therapy. After a femoral nerve deficit was observed in one patient, thin lead shields have routinely been placed over the psoas muscles during intra-operative therapy to protect the femoral nerve. Since then no similar problems have occurred. The cases of severe lumbar plexus neuropathy and ureteric obstruction were complications of radiation therapy from necrosis and fibrosis of the pelvic sidewall, and each required re-operation.

The high mortality and morbidity that occurred in this study indicates the need for additional basic investigation in animal models to determine the biological effects of high-dose intra-operative therapy, particularly when used in conjunction with conventional postoperative irradiation. Vascular and neural tissues cannot be moved from the treatment field and are at risk of serious injury when large cumulative doses are employed. Pelvic necrosis and fibrosis can lead to urinary tract obstruction, abscess formation and sepsis. Most clinical studies of intra-operative therapy used to treat other tumour sites have not used additional postoperative external beam treatment. This may explain the lower incidence of treatment-related mortality and morbidity previously described [5].

The rationale for investigating intra-operative radiotherapy in gynaecology is to improve tumour control relative to treatment complications. The results of this study demonstrate that although it appears to assist in the local control of a large tumour volume, a favourable effect on survival has not been demonstrated. The substantial treatment-related mortality and morbidity that occurred clearly indicates the need for further basic investigation to determine appropriate dose guidelines prior to future clinical studies.

References

1. Ballon S, Berman M, Lagasse L et al. (1981) Survival after extraperitoneal pelvic and para aortic lymphadenectomy and radiation therapy in cervical carcinoma. Obstet Gynecol 57:90–95
2. Abe M, Takahashi M (1981) Intraoperative radiotherapy: the Japanese experience. Int. J Radiat Oncol Biol Phys 7:863–868
3. Goldson A, Delgado G, Hill L (1978) Intraoperative radiation of the para-aortic nodes in cancer of the uterine cervix: Obstet Gynecol 52:713–717
4. Goldson A (1981) Past, present and prospects of intraoperative radiotherapy (IORT) Semin Oncol 8:59–64
5. Gunderson L, Tepper J, Biggs DJ et al (1983) Intraoperative and external beam radiation. Curr Probl. Cancer Vol 7(11):3–67
6. Sindelar WF, Kinsella T, Tepper J et al. (1983) Experimental and clinical studies with intraoperative radiotherapy. Surg Gynecol Obstet 157:205–219
7. Biggs P, Epp E, Ling C et al. (1981) Dosimetry, field shaping and other considerations for intraoperative electron therapy. Int J Radiat Oncol Biol Phys 7:875–884
8. Tepper J, Sindelar WF (1981) Summary of the workshop on intraoperative radiation therapy. Cancer Treat Rep 65:911–918

10 · Frozen Section Grading of Cervical Dysplasias in the Colposcopy Clinic: Audit and Appraisal

S.Fletcher, G.E.Smart and J.R.B.Livingstone*

Introduction

In the colposcopy clinic histological sections of cervical biopsies can be prepared rapidly by the freezing method and diagnosed immediately. Treatment (by laser, cold coagulator or cryocautery) can then be chosen rationally and completed at the same visit. By the paraffin method the extended processing entails discharging the patient, awaiting diagnosis, and recalling her for treatment often some weeks later. Immediate frozen section thus spares the patient considerable and prolonged anxiety.

To investigate the propriety of frozen sections as a diagnostic method we present a comparison of the influence of frozen and paraffin methods on the histological grading of cervical dysplasia.

The biopsies in the study were the first 282 (from 152 patients—Table 10.5) which the histopathologist (S.F.) reported by frozen section and they were cut on a cryostat which had seen long service. The frozen sections produced were more prone to disturbing artefacts than those from a machine in perfect order. Thus future technical refinements, bringing frozen sections closer to paraffin sections in legibility, might lead to better correlations than in the present survey.

* With the Statistical Assistance of Robert A. Elton, B.A. Ph.D., Senior Lecturer, Medical Computing and Statistics Unit, University of Edinburgh

Methods

Histological Techniques

Colposcopic cervical biopsies (average size 5 mm × 3 mm) were mounted in OCT embedding fluid (Tissue-Tek) on chucks, frozen by solid carbon dioxide, cut at a setting of 4 μm in the cryostat and stained by aqueous haemalum and eosin. Dehydrated and cleared sections were permanently mounted in Coverbond TM (Harleco) mounting medium and examined microscopically. An immediate report was given to the colposcopist.

The frozen blocks were thawed, fixed in formalin, and paraffin-embedded by technical staff. Permanent haemalum and eosin sections were prepared at a setting of 2 μm.

Grading Dysplasia

All gradings were carried out by the same pathologist (S.F.), whose previous experience was restricted to paraffin sections. The grades of Govan et al. [1] were used (Table 10.1) to give a six-point scale which was thought a more rigorous test of grading skills than the five-point scale [2]. In the presence of koilocytosis, dysplasia was referred to the same scale, as previously justified and illustrated [3]. Time was always allowed for the identity and grading of frozen sections to be forgotten before the corresponding paraffin gradings were carried out. Methods for recording the results prevented sight of the frozen grades until the paraffin grades had been entered.

Similarity of Sections

Paraffin and frozen sections from the same biopsy may differ markedly and were therefore classified as having 'similar', 'shared' or 'dissimilar' profiles. Comparison was aided by stacking the two slides and attempting superimposition of the sections at × 25 magnification under the stereoscopic microscope. Comparison was carried out in several attitudes, including inversion (mirror-imaging) of one section relative to the other.

Identification of Grading Surveys

For the comparisons two different surveys were carried out on the paired frozen and paraffin sections from each biopsy:

1. *First (diagnostic) grading*, which recorded the gradings first assigned to the sections *diagnostically* to determine the patient's treatment.
2. *Second (investigative) grading*, which helped to assess *within-observer variation on another occasion* 2–3 years after the first (diagnostic) survey.

Comparisons

Comparisons were carried out at two levels: (a) between the grades of *individual biopsies* and (b) between the *severest grades* found in all of the biopsies from one patient, i.e. the grades *determining the overall diagnosis* and the treatment.

Statistical Displays

The main instrument of comparison of the frozen and paraffin methods is the '6 × 6 square' as in Table 10.1. It segregates the observations which fall into each grade on frozen section (row total) into *each of the six grades* to which they were assigned on paraffin section. [Likewise, it segregates the number of observations in each grade on paraffin section (column total) into *each of the six grades* to which they were assigned on frozen section.] The properties of such arrays are sometimes ill-understood and a simplified introduction is prompted.

In the format used here the axes of the square carry the ordinal scales for the frozen and paraffin gradings, in increasing order of severity, from an origin at the top left hand corner (Table 10.1 and Fig. 10.1a).

Inspection confirms that the entries for numbers of observations sharing the same frozen and paraffin grades must fall in the grids which lie along the diagonal through the origin. A population with perfect frozen and paraffin correlation over all six grades would fill all the diagonal grids with its entries while all the others would be empty. Figure 10.1a depicts 'perfect' correlation by using shading for grids which bear entries. Figure 10.1b shows a distribution about the diagonal which is broader than perfection (each grade, by one method, is within ± 1 grade by the other method). It is a 'good' correlation (later we will examine the effects of variation in the *numbers* of entries in the grids, but for the present the assumption of an artificially uniform distribution in the shaded boxes will simplify matters).

'Perfect' and even 'good' correlations in natural populations are rare and entries are more usually broadly scattered (as in Table 10.1) and with different numerical values. Although at first sight a pattern may not be evident, statistical analysis and a knowledge of the extreme patterns of distribution are helpful in discerning trends. The two main and co-existing patterns of distribution are *bias* and *variability* of one grading method relative to the other.

Bias

In the context of graded severity of a lesion, bias can be specified as pessimism (or optimism) of one method relative to the other. For uniformity, only 'pessimism' is used here.

In Fig. 10.1c the occupied squares have shifted markedly into the lower triangle created by the main diagonal. When assessed by the frozen method there are many more occupied squares in the severer grades (4–6) than when assessed by paraffin. The frozen method is thus markedly more pessimistic in its bias than the paraffin.

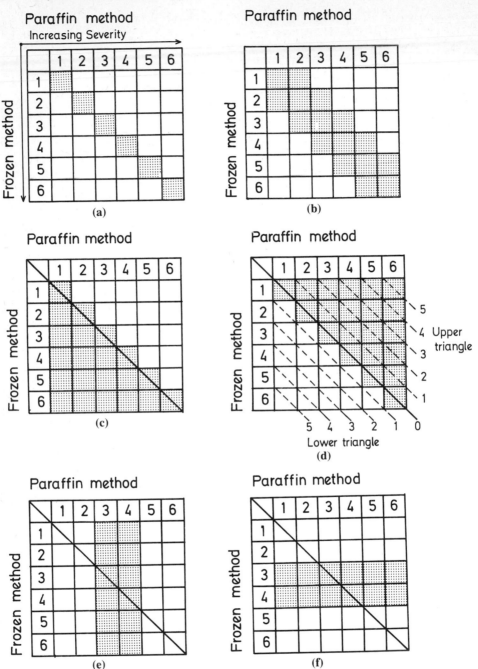

Fig. 10.1.a Perfect correlation. **b** 'Good' correlation. **c** Frozen method strongly pessimistic relative to paraffin. **d** Paraffin method strongly pessimistic relative to frozen. *Central diagonal (0)* creates a lower and upper triangle. Each *triangle* is divided by a numbered series *(1–5)* of corresponding diagonals. **e** 'Vertical' rectangular distribution of entries. Frozen method more variable than paraffin. **f** 'Horizontal' rectangular distribution of entries. Paraffin method more variable than frozen.

In general, relative shifts into the triangle which subtends the scale axis for a method renders that method more pessimistic relative to the other. Thus in Fig.10.1d the paraffin method is more pessimistic than the frozen method. However, the degree of pessimism is determined not only by the shape of the distribution, as in our artificial examples, but also by the *magnitude* of the entries in each box. Thus the entries in Fig.10.1b, which are presently assumed to be uniform, yield a symmetric distribution *without bias*. If, however, the entries in the grids along the lower edge were numerically substantially increased, then the distribution would indicate pessimism in the gradings by frozen section.

In practice, therefore, relative bias is usually very much less detectable (Table 10.1) than in the simple and extreme examples given and a display is needed which is more readily assimilable than the 6 × 6 square. The shift of entries into the upper and lower triangles can be gauged by the total numbers falling in each of the successive parallels to the central diagonal (as defined in Fig. 10.1d). The results (drawn from Table 10.1) can be arranged thus:

		Lower				Diagonal		Upper				
Axis	Sum	4	3	2	1	0	1	2	3	4	Sum	Axis
F>	108	2	3	22	81	133	32	7	2	0	41	>P

Direction of pessimism, frozen (F) > paraffin (P)

[Symbol F> -------------------- >P]

With some loss of information, the complex quadratic array of Table 10.1 has become a simple linear one in which entries in corresponding (equally weighted) diagonals can be compared readily and where the sums for each triangle are a crude measure of the strength and direction of pessimism.

Such 'reductionist' approaches are essential for assembling comprehensible displays allowing comparison of the content of several '6 × 6 squares'. Table 10.2 shows four such lines of figures summarising four parent 6 × 6 correlations each identified, along with its direction of pessimism, by symbols explained in the legend. The distributions change from one to another and the resulting directions and strength of pessimism are easy to compare.

Variability

Variability is the degree of spread of the entries through the available grades. Variability is defined as high when there is an even spread throughout the grades and low when there is clustering of entries in a few grades only, e.g. the central ones.

Figures 10.1e and 10.1f show the extreme case of a rectangular distribution of entries which is disposed vertically in Fig. 10.1e and horizontally in Fig.10.1f.

In Fig.10.1e the frozen method yields an even distribution throughout its six grades and is therefore *more variable* than the paraffin, where there is central clustering in grades 3 and 4, giving a very uneven distribution (*less variable*).

In Fig. 10.1f the paraffin method has the even distribution and is therefore *more variable* than the frozen.

Natural Distributions

Natural distributions in fact seldom conform to our extreme and simplified illustrations and usually fill most of the grids with numerical entries of different magnitude. Within the area occupied the location of the highest numerical values has the greatest effect on bias and variability according to the principles outlined in Fig. 10.1. The tendencies of the whole distribution can be separated and their significance measured by the non-parametric statistical methods quoted in the results [4].

Results

First (Diagnostic) Gradings of Frozen and Paraffin Sections Compared for Individual Biopsies

Table 10.1 compares the first (diagnostic) gradings of the paired frozen and paraffin sections: the scatter of biopsies away from the central diagonal of perfect correlation is evident.

The significance and direction of *pessimism* in the two methods were assessed by assembling (Table 10.2 line 1) the number of biopsies in successive parallels to the diagonal in the upper and lower triangles of Table 10.1. Table 10.2 (line 1) shows clearly the bias towards pessimism in all ranks of the triangle corresponding to the frozen gradings which is significant at $P < 0.001$ by the Wilcoxon signed-ranks test.

The *variability* of gradings—the tendency to wide distribution over all grades rather than to central clustering—is shown by extracting the row and column % totals from Table 10.1 and re-assembling them in Table 10.3. Here, lines 1 and 2 show a higher proportion of biopsies in the non-dysplastic and mild grades by the

Table 10.1. First (diagnostic) gradings: distribution of individual biopsies by frozen and paraffin methods

Frozen section gradings:	Paraffin section gradings						Row total (%)
	Non-dys.	Mild	Mod.	Sev.	C.i.S.	Inv.	
Non-dysplastic	26	1	4	1	0	0	32 (11.3)
Mild dysplasia	14	5	5	2	1	0	27 (9.6)
Moderate dysplasia	14	20	*12*	10	1	0	57 (20.2)
Severe dysplasia	3	3	18	*30*	16	0	70 (24.8)
Carcinoma-in-situ	2	0	5	29	*54*	0	90 (31.9)
Invasion	0	0	0	0	0	*6*	6 (2.1)
Column total	59	29	44	72	72	6	282
%	20.9	10.3	15.6	25.5	25.5	2.1	100

Table 10.2. Direction and significance of pessimism in grading; different surveys and methods compared. Distribution of individual biopsies in the lower and upper triangles of 6 × 6 squares arranged by diagonals

Vertical axis	Lower					Diagonal 0	Upper				Sum	Horizontal axis	Probability*
	Sum	4	3	2	1		1	2	3	4			
F1>	108	2	3	22	81	133	32	7	2	0	41	>P1	<0.001
F2>	70	0	3	14	53	170	38	5	0	1	44	>P2	<0.01
F1>	109	0	0	16	93	145	23	3	2	0	28	>F2	<0.001
P1>	72	0	1	10	61	169	35	5	1	0	41	>P2	<0.05

Key: F, frozen method; P, paraffin method; 1, first (or diagnostic) grading; 2, second (or investigative) grading. Direction of pessimism thus:
F1> ------------ >P1
* Wilcoxon signed-ranks test

Table 10.3. Variability of gradings: different surveys and methods compared. Distribution as percentages of individual biopsies

Pair compared	Non-dysplastic	Mild	Moderate	Severe	Carcinoma in situ	Invasion	Variability	Probability*
F1[a]	11.3	9.6	20.2	24.8	31.9	2.1	P1 > F1	<0.001
P1[a]	20.9	10.3	15.6	25.5	25.5	2.1		
F2	14.5	13.5	18.8	35.1	16.0	2.1	P2 > F2	<0.001
P2	24.6	8.1	18.2	27.7	18.6	2.8		
F1	11.3	9.6	20.2	24.8	31.9	2.1	–	NS
F2	14.5	13.5	18.8	35.1	16.0	2.1		
P1	20.9	10.3	15.6	25.5	25.5	2.1	–	NS
P2	24.1	7.8	18.4	28.0	18.8	2.8		

[a] Figures compiled from the row and column totals of Table 10.1 (percentages)
* Kendall rank correlation of sum versus difference

paraffin method than by the frozen method (significant at $P < 0.001$ by the Kendall rank correlation of sum versus difference). The paraffin method thus encourages greater variability or scatter by the reporter than does the frozen method, where there is relative clustering in the moderate to carcinoma-in-situ grades.

Second (Investigative) Gradings of Frozen and Paraffin Sections Compared for Individual Biopsies

A 6×6 square for the second (investigative) grading is not given but its derivatives are entered in Tables 10.2 and 10.3 as before. The results parallel the first gradings with some differences.

The relative bias towards *pessimism* is still evident in the frozen gradings (Table 10.2, line 2), the difference reaching significance at a probability of < 0.01. The correlation between frozen and paraffin gradings is thus slightly better on second grading.

Table 10.3 (lines 3 and 4) shows that the greater relative *variability* of paraffin gradings established in the first survey is also seen on the second at the same level of probability ($P < 0.001$).

The results of the first survey are thus resistant to substantial change at the second.

Within-Observer Difference: The Same Biopsy Twice Graded

More information on within-observer difference and the influence of frozen sections and paraffin sections upon it comes from comparisons of the first (diagnostic) and second (investigative) gradings of the *same* sections.

The results were essentially similar for both the frozen and paraffin methods:

Pessimism was always greatest on the first grading for either the frozen method (Table 10.2, line 3) or the paraffin method (line 4). The degree of pessimism, however, reached greater significance with the frozen method ($P < 0.001$) than with the paraffin ($P < 0.05$).

Variability did not show a significant difference between the first and second grading either for frozen sections (Table 10.3, lines 5 and 6) or for paraffin sections (lines 7 and 8).

Observer differences are thus insufficient to alter significantly the *variability* of the first and second gradings but sufficient to render the first (diagnostic) opinion more *pessimistic* than the second by both methods.

Influence of Similarity of Profiles of Frozen and Paraffin Sections

A major reason for the difference in gradings of a frozen section and its corresponding paraffin section is that they are never *strictly* identical. At best, and infrequently, the paraffin section may be parallel to the frozen section and several microns deeper, but usually the uncertainty of embedding yields random planes devoid of common features. Pairs of frozen and paraffin sections were classified as similar, shared (part of their profiles in common) or dissimilar in shape. The degree of correlation between the gradings of the frozen and paraffin sections in each group was calculated by Kendall's rank correlation.

Both the first and second gradings of the frozen and paraffin sections (Table 10.4, lines 1 and 2) show a clear downward trend in their correlation coefficients with increasing dissimilarity. A reasonable resemblance in the paired sections thus favours a like dysplastic grade in both.

Controls for the conclusions come from the first and second gradings of the frozen sections, and of the paraffin sections in the three groups (Table 10.4, lines 3 and 4). A trend in their correlation coefficients is not evident.

Table 10.4. Influence of face identity on correlation coefficients*. Figures based on individual biopsies

Comparison	Face identity		
	Similar	Shared	Dissimilar
F1 and P1	0.77	0.65	0.65
F2 and P2	0.85	0.77	0.70
F1 and F2	0.78	0.81	0.71
P1 and P2	0.84	0.63	0.77
n	68	26	188
%	24	9	67

*   Kendall rank correlation coefficient

Comparison of Frozen and Paraffin Methods for Severest Gradings

Patients often had multiple biopsies (Table 10.5) and only the severest grade determined treatment. Even with low averages (1.8 biopsies per patient) a comparison of the severest grades by frozen and paraffin methods from each patient might be expected to give closer correlations than those based on individual biopsies due to the number of samples yielding the severest grade.

The 'severest grades' of the 152 patients by both the frozen and the paraffin methods were thus extracted and statistically compared in the same format as Table 10.1 and in the same pairs as Tables 10.2 and 10.3. However, detailed data for the comparisons are not presented. Their trends and significance levels only are given later in Tables 10.9 and 10.10, where the overall conclusions of the whole study are collected.

Presumptive Wart Virus (Koilocytic) Lesions

Lesions of condyloma acuminatum were recorded in both surveys and the koilocytic state of the cervical biopsies was recorded in the second survey only.

Table 10.5. Number of biopsies per patient

Number of biopsies/patient	1	2	3	4	5	Total
Number of patients	54	69	27	1	1	152
Number of biopsies	54	138	81	4	5	282
Average biopsies per patient = 1.86						

Flat Koilocytosis in Dysplastic and Non-dysplastic States

Koilocytosis was merely recorded as absent or present in the section graded for dysplasia. Accordingly, koilocytosis should be regarded only as an accompaniment of the quoted degree of dysplasia. The intensity of koilocytosis and its precise relationship to the zones of quoted dysplasia, to any lesser grades, or to non-dysplastic epithelium accompanying it were not recorded. Dysplastic and koilocytic states for 282 biopsies are given for both the frozen and the paraffin method in Table 10.6.

The conclusions are:

1. Both the frozen and the paraffin methods confirm the progressive fall previously illustrated [3] in the incidence of koilocytosis in the severer dysplastic grades.

2. There is a significantly higher incidence of koilocytosis ($P < 0.001$, McNemar's test) by the paraffin method (48.6%) than by the frozen method (36.5%).

3. Frozen sections showed significantly more pessimistic grades in the group lacking koilocytes compared with that in which they were present (Wilcoxon rank sum test: $P < 0.01$). With the paraffin method a significant difference was not evident.

Thus, when grading by the frozen method, koilocytosis confers an optimistic bias. The significant effect of koilocytosis on the bias of the frozen grading suggested that there might also be an effect on the agreement between frozen and paraffin gradings. Table 10.7 gives comparisons of different combinations of subgroups by method and by the presence or absence of koilocytosis, for which the Kendall rank correlation coefficients are calculated.

For all combinations of koilocytic states the coefficients fail to establish a significant disturbance of the correlation between the frozen and paraffin grades obtained in the second (investigative) survey. The method used for grading dysplasia in the presence of koilocytes [3] therefore agrees well with the conventional method of grading dysplasia in their absence.

Plenary Koilocytosis

Plenary koilocytosis, or 'full thickness' koilocytosis, an uncommon state [3], was found in only 3 of 282 biopsies (1%). In two, the plenary state was accompanied by discrete foci of gradable non-koilocytic dysplasia (severe). In one other, the plenary state prevailed and was itself graded arbitrarily as moderate in the days before its grading was proscribed in favour of surveillance [3].

Table 10.6. Second (investigative) survey: koilocytosis and dysplastic grades

Method	Koilocytosis	Non-dys		Mild		Moderate		Severe		Carcinoma in situ		Invasion		Total	
		n	%	n	%	n	%	n	%	n	%	n	%	n	%
Frozen	Present	12	29%	21	55%	24	45%	38	38%	8	18%	0	0%	103	36.5%
	Absent	29	71%	17	45%	29	55%	61	62%	37	82%	6	100%	179	63.5%
Paraffin	Present	23	34%	13	59%	34	65%	47	59%	19	36%	1	12.5%	137	48.6%
	Absent	45	66%	9	41%	18	35%	32	41%	34	64%	7	87.5%	145	51.4%

Table 10.7. Second (investigative) survey: correlations between frozen and paraffin gradings in groups of biopsies with different koilocytic states

Koilocytosis in Frozen	Paraffin	Kendall rank correlation coefficient	n
Absent	Absent	0.74	116
Absent	Present	0.73	63
Present	Absent	0.60	29
Present	Present	0.75	74

Condyloma Acuminata

In the first survey condyloma acuminata was regarded as the prime diagnosis and was not qualified by attempts to grade dysplasia either within or without its boundaries. A total of seven (2.5%) condylomata were encountered, all paired in the frozen and paraffin sections.

In the second survey the numbers remained 7 (2.5%) by the frozen method and increased to 11 (3.8%) by the paraffin method. The increases reflect increased ability to detect a lesion which can easily escape recognition. Both methods give a majority of condyloma not associated with dysplasia (Table 10.8). Paraffin sections show a scatter of accompanying dysplastic grades which can be found both within and without the confines of the condyloma.

Table 10.8. Second (investigative) survey: individual biopsies with diagnosis of condyloma acuminatum

Method	Without dysplasia	With dysplasia: Mild	Moderate	Severe	C.i.S.	Total
Frozen	5	1	0	1	0	7
Paraffin	7	1[a]	1	1	1[a]	11

[a]   Dysplasia *within* the condyloma: other entries refer to dysplasia in the accompanying epithelium.

Discussion

Frozen section as a determinant of immediate treatment or as the sole diagnostic method is best examined relative to the confirmatory paraffin section in stringent conditions. Here, inexperience of frozen section reporting and sections cut on a well-worn cryostat and relatively difficult to read provided a measure of adversity which was further enhanced by making the conclusive comparisons at 'individual biopsy' level rather than at 'severest biopsy' or 'patient diagnosis' level.

The main findings of the study, including those derived from 'severest grades' not previously detailed but necessary for the final conclusions, are collected in Tables 10.9 and 10.10 and discussed below.

Table 10.9. Grading of dysplasia by frozen and paraffin methods. Influence on pessimism and variability

| Survey | Population compared | Grading property: | |
		Pessimism*	Variability[a]
First (diagnostic)	Individual biopsies	F1>P1 (<0.001)	P1>F1 (<0.001)
	Severest grading	F1>P1 (<0.01)	P1>F1 (<0.01)
Second (investigative)	Individual biopsies	F2>P2 (<0.01)	P2>F2 (<0.001)
	Severest grading	F2 = P2 (NS)	P2>F2 (<0.001)

Notation as in Table 10.2.
* Wilcoxon signed-ranks test.
[a] Kendall rank correlation of sum versus difference.

Table 10.10. Within-observer difference for pessimism and variability on regrading the same section (between diagnostic and investigative gradings). For 'individual biopsies' and 'severest gradings per patient'

| Population | Frozen method | | Paraffin method | |
	Pessimism*	Variability*	Pessimism*	Variability*
Individual biopsies	F1>F2 (<0.001)	F1 = F2 (NS)	P1>P2 (<0.05)	P1 = P2 (NS)
Severest grading	F1>F2 (<0.001)	F1 = F2 (NS)	P1 = P2 (NS)	P1 = P2 (NS)

* Notation as in Table 10.9.

Comparisons of 'Individual Biopsies'

In this section references to Tables 10.9 and 10.10 are *to the figures in the 'individual biopsy' rows only*, which give the most stringent comparisons of grading.

1. The *first (diagnostic) survey* (Table 10.9, line 1) is the most relevant to patient care and the frozen method gives significantly more *pessimistic* gradings than the paraffin. The paraffin method also shows significantly greater *variability*, or distribution throughout the grades, than the frozen method, where (details in Table 10.3, lines 1 and 2) there is a tendency to central clustering of entries which is less evident with the paraffin method.

The differences in *variability* may be explained by thinner, 'more readable' or 'clearer' paraffin sections which may promote greater discrimination between the grades. Relative to the paraffin method, diagnostic grading by frozen section certainly leads to a reluctance to use the 'non-dysplastic' category (Table 10.3, lines 1 and 2) while 'carcinoma-in-situ' is used a little more. Both tendencies also contribute to the significant *pessimism* of the frozen section gradings.

2. The *second (investigative) survey* provides data for several conclusions about changes in grading skills with time, which are well known to be significant [5].

Compared with the first (diagnostic) survey, *variability* in the frozen versus paraffin comparison remains the same (Table 10.9, lines 1 and 3) but the difference in *pessimism*, which still remains greater by the frozen method than by the paraffin, shows a reduced significance, i.e. the correlation is somewhat better. Changes in the observer's grading between surveys are not serious but merit further study:

3. *Within-Observer differences between surveys* which arise when *the same* frozen or paraffin section is graded twice are of interest as a guide to the reproducibility of grading and, in particular, to the changes in reporting pattern with increasing experience of frozen sections over 2–3 years.

Pessimism shows an interesting and strong relationship with the diagnostic process and with the frozen method.

Table 10.10 (line 1) shows that both the frozen method and the paraffin method give significantly more pessimistic gradings in the first (diagnostic) survey compared with the second (investigative) one. The difference with the frozen method is more significant and its strength is also shown by its persistence at undiminished significance into the 'severest gradings' comparison (line 2) whereas that of the paraffin method is reduced to nil.

Two hypotheses may separately or together explain the phenomenon: (a) The responsibility of diagnostic (first) grading may be relatively greater than the investigative (second) grading and may therefore confer a pessimistic bias by either method. The additional stress of reporting and determining treatment in the clinic may cause the diagnostic frozen grading to be significantly more pessimistic than the diagnostic paraffin grading. (b) In the 2–3 years between surveys the grading habits of the reporter may have altered only slightly for paraffin reporting but considerably for frozen reporting (due to increasing experience with it). The hypothesis is in keeping with the unfamiliarity of frozen section reporting and hence the greater opportunity for change. In contrast, the long previous experience of paraffin reporting would be less susceptible to change.

Whatever the reason it is clear that significant *pessimism* is related to the *diagnostic frozen section*.

Variability (Table 10.10 line 1) shows differences not reaching significance between the first (diagnostic) survey and the second (investigative) survey for both the frozen and the paraffin method. Thus, certain components of the grading skills have not changed between the surveys.

4. *Similarity of Frozen and Paraffin Sections:* Only 24% of section faces were 'similar' and strictly speaking comparisons are often between the incomparable. A reasonable resemblance between frozen and paraffin sections (Table 10.4) was found to favour a similar grade in both. The multiple, patchy nature of dysplasia and pre-selection by colposcopy probably account for the quite good correlations which are found in the 'dissimilar' population which account for 67% of the total in Table 10.4.

5. *Koilocytosis:* This was present in 36.5% of frozen sections and 48.6% of paraffin sections from the biopsies studied (including the non-dysplastic grade). The much higher incidence of koilocytes by the paraffin method could be due to a number of properties: thinner, more 'readable' sections facilitating their detection, preparative shrinkage increasing their density per unit volume of section, and dehydration and vacuum embedding causing some artefactual production.

Koilocytosis conferred an optimistic bias on gradings by the frozen method but did not significantly influence the paraffin gradings. Plenary koilocytosis [3] was confirmed to be rare (1%).

6. *Condyloma Acuminata:* Slightly increased numbers of condyloma acuminata found in the second survey suggest that it easily escapes detection, especially in its early stages, when biopsies are small or the plane of section fails to show exophytic processes. The colposcopist is best placed to recognise early condyloma acu-

minata and should always alert the pathologist to the probability. Dysplasia may not be detected unless biopsies are taken from both the condylomatous and the non-condylomatous areas. Histologically, planes of section tangential to the hyperplastic basal zones of the acanthotic processes of condyloma acuminata can suggest alarming degrees of dysplasia. Later review of the solitary case of 'severe' dysplasia within a condyloma (Table 10.8) suggested that the dysplasia was of lesser degree (moderate to mild).

Comparisons of 'Severest Grading'

The severest grading found among all the cervical biopsies taken from a patient was always quoted as the final diagnosis.

Comparisons of 'severest gradings' show a general resemblance to those for 'individual biopsies' but the differences between frozen and paraffin distributions are less significant, or more congruent.

The effect is seen (with one unimportant exception) throughout Table 10.9, where the most practically relevant figure is that for the pessimism of the first (diagnostic) frozen grading relative to its paraffin. It is significantly reduced when compared at the level of 'severest grading'.

Observer differences between the two surveys of the same section (by either method) are given in Table 10.10. Here, variability for the 'individual biopsies' comparison is already not significant by both methods: making the same comparisons at 'severest grading' level is without further effect.

Pessimism, however, for the paraffin method shows a fall in the significance of the difference between the two surveys when the comparison is changed from 'individual biopsies' to 'severest grading'.

Even with an average of 1.8 biopsies per patient the improved congruence with 'severest grade' comparisons suggests that, within limits, an increase in the number of selective biopsies per patient would both increase the detection of dysplasia and shift the final frozen diagnosis in the direction of a paraffin report.

Conclusion

Tested in adversity frozen sections relative to paraffin give more pessimistic diagnostic gradings of cervical dysplasia. Although the bias of the frozen method may determine some unnecessary treatment of non-dysplastic states (by laser), overdiagnosis of invasion was not encountered (Table 10.1). As tested, we find it a safe determinant of immediate treatment. Improved technique, increasing experience and the effect of multiple biopsies can only improve the correlation with the paraffin method.

An account of our experience with it, of improved methods and of its many advantages in colposcopic training and research is in preparation.

Summary

A single observer compared the dysplastic gradings of his first 282 frozen sections of cervix with those of their paired paraffin sections on two occasions, one *diagnostic*, the other, after 2–3 years, *investigative*:

1. Both the frozen method (relative to the paraffin) and the diagnostic grading (relative to the investigative) confer pessimism on dysplastic gradings which is most significant in a 'diagnostic frozen section'.
2. Paraffin gradings show greater variability (scatter) throughout the grades whereas frozen gradings cluster centrally.
3. The within-observer difference between diagnostic and investigative gradings on the *same* section shows that neither method confers significant variability. The diagnostic grading by both methods is more pessimistic than the investigative.
4. Multiple biopsies from one patient are reported as the 'severest grading' and when compared at that level (rather than as 'individual biopsies') the differences between frozen and paraffin gradings are reduced significantly.
5. Only 24% of paired frozen and paraffin sections have similar profiles. Resemblance favours a similar grading.
6. Koilocytosis was significantly more frequent in paraffin sections (49%) than in frozen sections (37%). It confers an optimistic bias on frozen gradings, none on paraffin gradings.
7. Early condyloma acuminatum will escape detection less often if the colposcopist's suspicions are conveyed to the pathologist.

References

1. Govan ADT, Haines RM, Langley FA, Taylor CW, Woodcock AS (1969) The history and cytology of changes in the epithelium of the cervix uteri. J Clin Pathol 22:383–395
2. Richart RM (1973) Cervical intraepithelial neoplasia: a review. Pathol Annu 8:301–328
3. Fletcher S (1983) Histopathology of papilloma virus infection of the cervix uteri: the history, taxonomy, nomenclature and reporting of koilocytic dysplasia. J Clin Pathol 36:616–624
4. Siegel S (1956) Nonparametric statistics for the behavioural sciences. McGraw-Hill, London
5. Cocker J, Fox H, Langley FA (1968) Consistence in the histological diagnosis of epithelial abnormalities of the cervix uteri. J Clin Pathol 21 67–70

Endometrium

11 · Biochemical and Morphological Effects of Oestrogen/Progestin Therapy on the Endometrium of Postmenopausal Women

W. E. Gibbons and D. Moyer

Introduction

Postmenopausal oestrogen replacement therapy has enjoyed a varied reputation and acceptance over the past decade. Its value for treatment of vasomotor flushing and thinning of urogenital tissues was recognised early. It was years later before there was sufficient experience to attest to the positive role of oestrogen therapy in the prevention of osteoporosis. In the United States the role of oestrogen replacement therapy was irreversibly altered with the observation that exogenous oestrogen use was associated with adenocarcinoma of the endometrium [1,2]. Subsequently, the use of oestrogens in the menopause began to decline. The relationship of oestrogen administration and the progressive development of abnormal endometrial histology has been shown by Paterson to be both dose and duration dependent [3]. By following endometrial biopsies at 6 month intervals, Paterson noted that as the concentration and potency of the oestrogen stimulus increased so did the incidence of abnormal endometrial histology. These changes could be antagonised by the administration of a progestin. Further, if the duration of the progestin administration was 10 days or greater, no abnormalities of the endometrial histology were noted. This suggested a duration effect of the progestin use as well.

Even though progestins antagonise the effects of oestrogens on endometrial growth, they do not antagonise the benefits of oestrogen therapy. Schiff has shown that progestins by themselves can reduce vasomotor flushing [4]. Judd et al. have also shown that oral medroxyprogesterone acetate can reduce urinary calcium loss [5]. Importantly, Christiansen's data suggest that there is a synergistic effect between the oestrogen and progestin that may result in an increase in bone mineral content [6], an effect only seen with high doses of oral oestrogen [7].

Whitehead et al. have shown that 19-nortestosterone progestins effectively antagonise the biochemical effects of nuclear accumulation of oestrogen receptor, a measure of oestrogen activity, and thymidine labelling, which is an index of cellular mitotic activity [8]. However, the 19-nortestosterones appear to lower serum levels of high-density lipoproteins (HDL) which potentially might increase the risk of arteriosclerotic heart disease [9]. This adverse affect is not noted with medroxyprogesterone acetate. We therefore evaluated the effects of different concentrations of medroxyprogesterone acetate on the endometrial parameters of histology and oestrogen receptor concentrations in postmenopausal women receiving different dosages of conjugated equine oestrogens [10].

Method

Three groups of postmenopausal women were given either 0.3 mg, 0.625 mg or 1.25 mg of conjugated equine oestrogen per day. There were five women in the two higher oestrogen dosage groups and three in the 0.3 mg oestrogen group. The average age of the women was 57 years and all were within twenty percent of their ideal body weight. Baseline oestrone and oestradiol levels were in the menopausal range and pretreatment endometrial biopsies revealed atropic changes.

Each oestrogen dosage group underwent four treatment cycles consisting of 25 days of oestrogen therapy. The four treatment cycles were separated by a 4-week interval on no therapy. The first treatment cycle consisted of oestrogen alone. The second cycle consisted of 25 days of oestrogen therapy plus 2.5 mg medroxyprogesterone acetate (Provera) administered on oestrogen treatment days 15–25. The third treatment cycle consisted of oestrogen plus 5 mg of medroxyprogesterone acetate (days 15–25). In the fourth cycle the pattern was the same except that 10 mg medroxyprogesterone acetate was administered.

On the 25th day of oestrogen administration in each of the four treatment cycles, the women underwent endometrial biopsy for histological evaluation and determination of cytosolic and nuclear oestrogen receptor content. For histological sections the biopsy tissue was placed in formalin, dehydrated and blocked in paraffin sections. An endometrial biopsy was obtained 4 weeks after the last treatment cycle to document endometrial histology before patients were discharged from the study.

For receptor analysis the tissues were washed and placed in ice-cold, isotonic buffer (10 mM Tris, 1.5 mM EDTA, 12 mM thioglycerol and 10% glycerol). The oestrogen receptor studies were performed as described in a previous publication [11] by a micro-assay technique utilising hydroxyapatite to separate bound from free hormone. Correlation coefficients were determined by regression analysis.

Results

Receptor Measurement

By determining the difference between the baseline, pre-treatment cytosol levels and the oestrogen-alone, stimulated cytosol level in each subject-matched pair of samples, a relationship was determined for the level of oestrogen receptor in the cytosol and the amount of oestrogen administered (Fig. 11.1). This response was linear with a correlation coefficient of 0.99.

The addition of 2.5 mg medroxyprogesterone acetate to the oestrogen treatment cycles resulted in a suppression of cytosolic oestrogen receptor to levels seen in the untreated samples (Fig. 11.2) from women receiving 0.3 mg and 0.625 mg of conjugated oestrogens, but not in those patients receiving 1.25 mg per day. Both 5 and 10 mg of the progestin were capable of suppressing the cytosolic oestrogen receptor levels to baseline levels in all oestrogen treatment groups. When nuclear levels of oestrogen receptor were compared (Fig. 11.3), antagonism of oestrogen receptor accumulation was seen for all medroxyprogesterone acetate dosages.

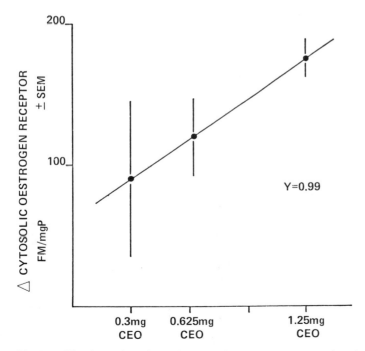

Fig. 11.1. The change in endometrial oestrogen receptor concentration observed in postmenopausal women when placed on various dosages of conjugated equine oestrogens (*CEO*).

CYTOSOLIC OESTROGEN RECEPTOR

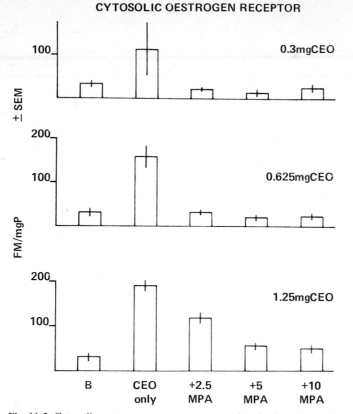

Fig. 11.2. Cytosolic oestrogen receptor concentrations in the endometrium of postmenopausal women on no therapy (*B*), conjugated equine oestrogens (*CEO*) or on conjugated oestrogens plus various dosages (in mg) of medroxyprogesterone acetate (*+MPA*).

Histology

Each endometrial biopsy specimen was evaluated for the following parameters: gland epithelial height, gland diameter, glands showing secretion (percent), quality of secretion, pseudodecidual stroma and subnuclear vacuoles (percent). The histological patterns of all pre-treatment biopsies revealed atrophic endometrium as did all biopsies performed 4 weeks after the last treatment cycle. Only minimal oestrogenic change was observed in the 0.3 mg oestrogen group, while marked oestrogenic stimulation occurred with the 0.625 mg and 1.25 mg oestrogen-only biopsies.

When medroxyprogesterone acetate was added to the oestrogen therapy, the morphological effects varied with the dose. None of the endometrial biopsies taken from women on 2.5 mg medroxyprogesterone acetate demonstrated a progestational response. Because of their biochemical similarity, the 5 mg and 10 mg medroxyprogesterone acetate cycles were compared. There were three patients in the 0.625 mg estrogen group (Table 11.1) and four women in the 1.25 mg estrogen group (Table 11.2) in whom there was sufficient material to evaluate

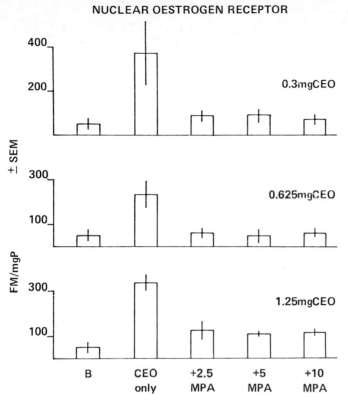

Fig. 11.3. Nuclear oestrogen receptor concentrations in the endometrium of postmenopausal women on no therapy (*B*), conjugated equine oestrogens (*CEO*), or on conjugated oestrogens plus various dosages (in mg) of medroxyprogesterone acetate (*+MPA*).

Table 11.1. Histological comparison of 5 mg and 10 mg of medroxyprogesterone acetate. 0.625 mg conjugated oestrogen

	5 mg	10 mg	*P* value
Gland epithelial height (μm)	17.33 ± 4.04	23.33 ± 7.64	<0.2
Gland diameter (μm)	63.33 ± 20.8	105 ± 35	<0.1
Per cent glands, showing			
secretion (%)	6.67 ± 5.77	50 ± 14.14	<0.05
Quality of secretion (+)	0.5 ± 0.5	2.16 ± 1.76	<0.1
Pseudodecidual stroma (+)	0 ± 0	1.13 ± 1.15	<0.1
Subnuclear vacuoles (%)	5 ± 7.07	1 ± 1.41	

n = 3

all of the morphologic parameters. However, in both oestrogen dosage groups the progestagenic response of 10 mg medroxyprogesterone acetate was always higher than that of 5 mg. Further, 10 mg medroxyprogesterone acetate promoted a more homogeneous secretory change in the stroma and glands than the more focal change noted with the 5 mg dose.

Table 11.2. Histological comparison of 5 mg and 10 mg of medroxyprogesterone acetate. 1.25 mg conjugated oestrogen

	5 mg	10 mg	P value
Gland epithelial height (μm)	23.5 ± 4.43	35.75 ± 9.95	<0.05
Gland diameter (μm)	91.25 ± 27.5	127.5 ± 35.71	<0.1
Per cent glands, showing			
secretion (%)	42.5 ± 27.2	88.75 ± 9.46	<0.01
Quality of secretion (+)	2 ± 1.08	3.5 ± 0.58	<0.025
Pseudodecidual stroma (+)	0.875 ± 1.44	2.5 ± 1.0	<0.1
Subnuclear vacuoles (%)	13.75 ± 7.50	3.75 ± 1.50	<0.1

$n = 4$

Discussion

From a risk/benefit point of view the most defensible reason for administering oestrogens to a postmenopausal woman on a long-term basis is the prevention of osteoporosis. Epidemiological evidence suggests that those who are at high risk for osteoporotic bone fractures include: fair-skinned or light-weight persons, smokers, heavy drinkers, those with early menopause, etc. [12]. Negative associations for hip fracture include: oestrogen replacement therapy, intact ovaries, and weight [13]. Hip fracture patients appear to have lower ideal body weights and higher concentrations of serum sex hormone binding globulin, which results in lower concentrations of biologically available oestradiol and testosterone [14]. Subsequently, it has been shown that exogenous oestrogens can prevent loss of bone mineral content [15] and 0.625 mg of conjugated equine oestrogens every day orally appears to result in urinary calcium/creatinine ratios that are in the premenopausal range [16]. Lindsay et al. have recently reported that conjugated equine estrogens in doses of 0.625 mg and 1.25 mg per day were equally effective in reducing bone loss as evaluated by single-photon absorptiometry, but dose levels less than 0.625 were ineffective [17].

The route of administration of the oestrogen may be oral, by subcuticular implant, transdermal or vaginal. The subcuticular implants may result in the highest levels of continuous oestrogen stimulation of the endometrium [3] and breast [18], and may pose the highest risk of neoplastic change. A transdermal route, such as oestradiol-containing gel, offers the apparent advantages over oral administration of reduced conversion to the less active oestrone and the metabolic advantage of reduced stimulation of oestrogen-sensitive lipoproteins [19]. However, the long-term efficacy on reduction of calcium loss still requires clarification [20]. The vaginal route can similarly deliver effective local and adequate systemic oestrogenic stimulation but, at least for the conjugated oestrogens, requires a higher dose on a per weight basis than the oral form for equivalent effect [21].

The widespread use of oestrogen replacement therapy in the postmenopausal woman leads to observation of its relationship to the development of carcinoma of the endometrium [2]. This risk has been shown by Gambrell and others to be effectively minimised by the concurrent use of a progestin [22]. Gambrell reports that the addition of a progestin to oestrogen replacement can reduce the risk to below that expected for women on no oestrogen replacement. Perhaps of even greater significance is Gambrell's report that the use of progestin postmenopausally may markedly reduce the incidence of breast cancer [23]. The protective effect on endometrium appears to be dose related, with greater benefit shown when the duration of progestin use in each cycle exceeds 10 days. This mirrors the short-term results of Paterson on endometrial histology after oestrogen stimulation quoted earlier [3]. The choice of progestin is still controversial. The 19-nortestosterone compounds such as norethindrone are effective in antagonising the oestrogenic stimulation of the endometrium [8], but appear to reduce the high density lipoprotein levels that might increase the risk of ischaemic heart disease [24]. This does not seem to be the case for natural progesterone or medroxyprogesterone acetate.

In our study there was a disparity between the biochemical and morphological results. Even though 5 mg and 10 mg of medroxyprogesterone acetate behaved identically in antagonising increases in cytosolic oestrogen receptor, 10 mg was superior by morphological criteria. Further, the progestational change seen with the 10 mg dose resulted in a more homogeneous change, whereas the effect of 5 mg medroxyprogesterone acetate was more focal in nature. The data on long-term administration of 5 mg medroxyprogesterone acetate on abnormal endometrial histology, including adenocarcinoma, are lacking, but focal, non-homogeneous antagonism of oestrogen effect would not seem optimal.

The dissociation of the biochemical and endometrial events has been hinted at in the past. The biochemical data of Whitehead demonstrate a plateau of effect after 6 days of administration [8]. The epidemiological data, on the other hand, suggest that 7 days of therapy alone is insufficient to block abnormal histological changes completely [3,22].

What then would be the current recommendation for therapy? As administered by an oral route, in a cyclic fashion, it would appear that 0.625 mg of conjugated equine oestrogens is the present minimal dose for prevention of osteoporosis. A progestin should be added to all women on oestrogen replacement. The benefits of reduced neoplasia of breast and uterus along with synergistic effects on bone mineral content and vasomotor instability outweigh the inconvenience of withdrawal bleeding. A progestin should be administered for >10 days per oestrogen cycle. If medroxyprogesterone acetate is used then 10 mg daily is the lowest recommended dose.

In our study, minimum stimulation of the endometrium occurred with 0.3 mg of conjugated equine oestrogen. The effects of progestins on endometrial histology is biphasic. An initial acute effect demonstrates the conversion of the endometrium to a secretory pattern. More chronic exposure results in atrophic change. The synergistic effect of oestrogen/progestin on bone loss may allow further reduction of the minimum requirements for each. Combined administration thoughout a cycle may result in minimal stimulation of endometrial growth along with the atrophic affect of chronic progestin administration, which may result in no breakthrough bleeding. Preliminary trials of combination therapy are in progress.

Who should be treated? Therapy could be limited to symptomatic subjects or those at high risk for osteoporosis. However, with the suggestion that progestin therapy may reduce breast cancer risk and until there is a practical, objective method for determining those women who do not need hormonal replacement, the recommendation is that all women without contraindications to therapy should receive oestrogen/progestin therapy. The understanding and rationale for postmenopausal hormone replacement is still evolving. Thus, it can be expected that treatment recommendations will continue to be modified. It is important now that we recognise the benefits of oestrogen therapy, comprehend the risks rationally, and add a progestin to all who receive oestrogen replacement therapy.

References

1. Gray LA, Christopherson WM, Hoover RN (1977) Estrogens and endometrial carcinoma. Obstet Gynecol 49:385–389
2. Mack T, Pike M, Henderson B et al. (1976) Estrogens and endometrial cancer in a retirement community. N Engl J Med 294:1262–1267
3. Paterson ME, Wade-Evans T, Sturdee DW et al. (1980) Endometrial disease after treatment with oestrogens and progestins in the climacteric. Br Med J I:822–824
4. Schiff I (1982) The effects of progestins on vasomotor flushes. J Reprod Med 27:498–502
5. Mandel FP, Davidson BJ, Erlik Y et al. (1982) Effects of progestins on bone metabolism in postmenopausal women. J Reprod Med 27:511–514
6. Christiansen C, Christiansen MS, Transbol I (1981) Bone mass in postmenopausal women after withdrawal of oestrogen/gestagen replacement therapy. Lancet I:459–461
7. Horsman A, Jones M, Francis R et al. (1981) The effect of estrogen dose on postmenopausal bone loss. N Engl J Med 309:1405–1407
8. Whitehead MI, Townsend PT, Pryse-Davies J et al. (1981) Effects of estrogens and progestins on the biochemistry and morphology of the postmenopausal endometrium. N Engl J Med 305:1599–1605
9. Hirvonen E, Malkonen M, Manninen V (1981) Effects of different progestins on lipoproteins during postmenopausal replacement therapy. N Engl J Med 304:560–563
10. Gibbons WE, Moyer D, Roy S et al. (to be published) Biochemical and histological effects of combined estrogen/progestin therapy on the endometrium of postmenopausal women. Obstet Gynecol
11. Hung TT, Gibbons WE (1983) Evaluation of androgen antagonism of estrogen effect by dihydrotestosterone. J Steroid Biochem 19:1513–1520
12. Saville PD (1984) Postmenopausal osteoporosis and estrogens. Who should be treated and why? Postgrad Med 75:135–138
13. Dreiger N, Kelsey JL, Holford TR et al. (1982) An epidemiologic study of hip fractures in postmenopausal women. Am J Epidemiol 116:141–148
14. Davidson BJ, Ross RK, Paganini-Hill A et al. (1982) Total and free estrogens and androgens in postmenopausal women with hip fractures. J Clin Endocrinol Metab 54:115–120
15. Lindsay R, Hart DM, Aitken JM et al. (1976) Long-term prevention of postmenopausal osteoporosis by oestrogen. Evidence of an increased bone mass after delayed onset of oestrogen treatment. Lancet I:1038–1041
16. Geola FL, Frumar AM, Tataryn IV et al. (1980) Biological effects of various doses of conjugated equine estrogens in postmenopausal women. J Clin Endocrinol Metab 51:620–625
17. Lindsay R, Hart DM, Clark DM (1984) The minimum effective dose of estrogen for prevention of postmenopausal bone loss. Obstet Gynecol 63:759
18. Hulka BS, Chambless LE, Deubner DC, et al. (1982) Breast cancer and estrogen replacement therapy. Am J Obstet Gynecol 143:638–644
19. Holst J (1983) Percutaneous estrogen therapy. Endometrial response and metabolic effects. Acta Obstet Gynecol Scand [Suppl] 115:1–30
20. Laufer LR, DeFazio JL, Lu JK et al. (1983) Estrogen replacement by transdermal estradiol administration. Am J Obstet Gynecol 146:533–540
21. Mandel FP, Geola FL, Meldrum DR et al. (1983) Biological effects of various doses of vaginally administered conjugated equine estrogens in postmenopausal women. J Clin Endocrinol Metab 57:133–139

22. Gambrell RD Jr (1982) The menopause: Benefits and risks of estrogen-progestin replacement therapy. Fertil Steril 37:457
23. Gambrell RD Jr, Maier RC, Sanders BI (1983) Decreased incidence of breast cancer in postmenopausal estrogen–progestin users. Obstet Gynecol 62:435–443
24. Fahraeus L, Larsson-Cohn U, Wallentin L (1983) L-Norgestrel and progesterone have different influences on plasma lipoproteins. Eur J Clin Invest 13:447–453

12 · Hormonal Treatment of Gynaecological Tumours

J. Bonte

Introduction

In gynaecological cancer there is a good theoretical basis for the use of steroid hormones, particularly those of ovarian origin. Those organs which have developed from the Müllerian duct and the urogenital sinus, as well as the ovaries themselves, are considered to be target organs for oestrogen and progesterone both in their morphological development and in their maintenance of function. Furthermore, oestrogens may be involved in the formation of some primary cancers of the endometrium and breast, or their metastases and recurrences. Thus some endometrial adenocarcinomas and breast cancers are oestrogen-dependent and could therefore respond to the antagonistic influences of progestogens and anti-oestrogens. Moreover, tubal and cervical adenocarcinoma as well as endometrioid and mesonephroid ovarian carcinoma may respond to progestogens and anti-oestrogens in view of their common embryological and pathological background.

More recently, these theoretical grounds for hormone dependency and responsiveness of gynaecological malignancies have been substantiated by data provided by steroid receptor determination. The high oestrogen and progesterone cytosol receptor concentrations found in most endometrial carcinomas support the principle that endometrial adenocarcinoma is related to abnormal oestrogenic stimulation. This hormone-dependent cancer is used as a model for in vitro and in vivo evaluation of progestational and anti-oestrogenic treatment.

Effects of Progestogens and Anti-oestrogens on Endometrial Adenocarcinoma

Cytological Data

Progestogens inhibit tumour growth directly, both in vitro in human endometrial adenocarcinoma cell lines [1] and in chemically induced tumours in mice [2]. Moreover, this growth inhibition is dose dependent [1,3] and is characterised at a cellular level by normalisation of nuclear morphology, reappearance of hetero-chromatin [4], a significant fall of DNA content [5], and a decrease in polyploidy [6]. Medroxyprogesterone acetate (MPA), in concentrations of 20 µg/ml, has been found to inhibit mitosis in more than 85% of endometrial adenocarcinoma cell cultures, with no evidence of tumour stimulation.

Anti-oestrogens attack adenocarcinomatous cells by direct inhibition of mitosis. The mitotic index of endometrial adenocarcinoma cells, as measured by tritiated thymidine incorporation, is markedly reduced in more than 40% of the cultures by addition of tamoxifen 1–2 µg/ml to the medium. However, in 28% of the cases, tamoxifen seems to stimulate the mitotic index. These data fit with the explosive progression that is sometimes observed in vaginal recurrence of poorly differentiated endometrial adenocarcinoma following tamoxifen therapy.

Progestogens induce a rapid and significant fall of cytosol oestrogen receptor (ER) content in cancer cells, thus inhibiting DNA synthesis [7,8,9]. The rapid changes in oestrogen receptor levels suggest unmasking of receptors rather than synthesis and degradation, which would more likely be related to the cell cycle [10]. Progestogens also reduce the cytosol progesterone receptor (PR) content in endometrial adenocarcinoma, usually to an undetectable level [8,9]. The reasons for progesterone receptor disappearance involve nuclear translocation and non-replenishment of receptors [8]. This negative control of progesterone receptor levels may diminish the effect of long-term progestational treatment in endo-metrial adenocarcinoma.

These principles of steroid receptor manipulation can be applied to most endometrial adenocarcinomas treated by the administration of 150 mg MPA per day. Of oestrogen receptor positive adenocarcinomas, 75% present a decrease in receptor content, while tumours totally devoid of oestrogen receptors reveal no change at all. In all types of endometrial adenocarcinomas, MPA reduces pro-gesterone receptor content, probably by exhaustion of the cytosol reserve [11]. Anti-oestrogens inhibit tumour growth via cytosol and nuclear steroid receptors. In the target cell, and especially in the endometrial cell, tamoxifen inhibits the binding of oestradiol to the cytosol receptors, reduces the concentration of these receptors and interferes with replenishment of the cytosol receptors. In addition, there is evidence that tamoxifen stimulates progesterone receptor synthesis. Tamoxifen may exert a similar action on endometrial adenocarcinoma [12]. In practice, the steroid receptor variations induced by tamoxifen seem to depend on the original receptor concentration in the tumour cells. In endometrial adeno-carcinomas with a high oestrogen receptor content, 40 mg tamoxifen daily induces a decrease in oestrogen receptors after 7 days. In adenocarcinomas with low oestrogen receptor content, however, tamoxifen provokes an increase in receptors, while in adenocarcinomas without oestrogen receptors, it produces either no change or receptor synthesis. Tamoxifen induces synthesis or an increase of the progesterone receptors in 71% of adenocarcinoma cells devoid of progesterone receptor or with a low progesterone receptor content; it provokes an increase in only 33% of high progesterone receptor containing endometrial adenocarcinomas [11].

Histological Data

The histological response of endometrial adenocarcinoma to medroxy-progesterone is dependent on the differentiation of the tumour and is generally characterised by [13]:

Enhanced secretory activity, with formation of subnuclear vacuoles.

The transformation of pseudostratified cells to activate monolayered glands.

Marked epithelial metaplasia of some glandular structures, especially in adenoacanthomatous tumours.

Pseudodecidualisation of the stroma.

Atrophy of the epithelium and fibrosis of the stroma, leading to breakdown of the tumour substance.

The histochemical evaluation of endometrial adenocarcinoma treated with progestogens shows substantial accumulation of glycogen, glycoproteins and mucopolysaccharides in the cytoplasm [13,14]. The ultrastructural response of the adenocarcinomatous cells to progestational agents consists of secretory conversion, decrease in length of the microvilli and loss of the cilia [15].

At the normal dosage of 20 mg two or three times a day, tamoxifen induces different histological and histochemical transformations according to tumour differentiation. The pseudostratified glands of the moderately differentiated adenocarcinoma are rapidly transformed to monolayered structures consisting of high cylindrical and, later on, even atrophic cells. Well differentiated cancers show atrophy and even necrosis. All responsive tumours are characterised by decidualisation of their stroma. In contrast to the evident secretory activity induced by MPA, tamoxifen sometimes induces glycogen, seldom mucopolysaccharide accumulation [16].

Endocrinological Data

The absence of statistically significant changes in steroid hormone plasma levels under medium dosage medroxyprogesterone administration, makes an indirect mechanism for the action of progestogens on endometrial adenocarcinoma rather improbable. Administration of 1 g medroxyprogesterone weekly induces no significant changes in oestradiol and oestrone plasma concentrations.

In comparison with the endocrinological changes induced by medroxyprogesterone, a possible indirect mechanism of action of anti-oestrogens on endometrial adenocarcinoma seems to be more evident. Tamoxifen provokes a fall of luteinising hormone (LH) and prolactin [17], and a slight decrease of oestradiol and oestrone serum levels [16].

Vaginal cytology represents another method of assessing induced endocrinological changes. Medroxyprogesterone treatment is characterised by a shift
of the vaginal smear to atrophy, typically in those patients with hormone responsive adenocarcinomas. Under short-term tamoxifen treatment the vaginal smear
remains mostly oestrogenic. Long-term tamoxifen therapy induces a shift of the
vaginal smear to a level characteristic for a high or medium oestrogenic stimulation in 60% of patients. In only 35% does the vaginal smear remain unchanged.
This cytological change seems to occur irrespective of tumour response [18].

Clinical Data

In addition to progesterone, more than ten different progestogens have been used
in the treatment of endometrial adenocarcinoma, either by local intracavitary
application, medium dose oral or intramuscular administration [19].

Local intracavitary application of progestogens appears to be effective in the
eradication of invasive stage I endometrial adenocarcinoma. After intrauterine
instillation, the tumour completely disappeared in approximately 35% of the
cases. Intrauterine insertion of a MPA-releasing device achieves total destruction
of malignant tissue in 60% of uteri which had no myometrial invasion and, in that
way, is able to replace preoperative radium packing [20].

In approximately 60% of patients with in situ endometrial carcinoma treated
with systemic progestogens, no residual cancer can be detected. However, the
same progestational therapy completely destroys only 20% of invasive stage I
endometrial adenocarcinomas. Thus, systemic progestational therapy alone is
indicated in selected cases, such as carcinoma-in-situ of the endometrium in a
younger woman still intending to have children. Nevertheless, in stage I endometrial adenocarcinoma, progestogens may be used as adjuvant therapy to radiosurgical management of endometrial adenocarcinomas [21]. Progestogens are
administered prior to radium application or hysterectomy, or during the
postoperative period. This adjuvant therapy reduces markedly both the incidence
of residual tumour and the recurrence rate [19]. Moreover, the survival rates
prove to be higher in patients receiving adjuvant hormone therapy compared with
those in the control group [22,23]. In advanced (stages III and IV) and in
recurrent endometrial adenocarcinoma, progestogens are the treatment of choice
and can be used in combination with radiotherapy. An impressive number of
collaborative, individual and case reports published on the response of advanced
or recurrent endometrial adenocarcinoma to progestogens show a mean objective
remission rate of approximately 30%–35% [19,24]. The factors influencing
response in such cases can be divided into those related to the administration of
the progestational compound, and those related to the responsiveness of the
tumour and the host. Response to the progestational agent is conditioned by the
type of drug and its plasma levels, determined by dosage, route and duration of
administration. Comparison of the mean objective remission rates for the most
frequently used progestational compounds permits their listing in relation to
cancericidal effectiveness: progesterone 56%, MPA 35%–57%, megestrol 33%–
41%, megestrone 21%–34% and hydroxyprogesterone caproate 18%–33% [25].
Taking into account the difficulties of administering progesterone at sufficient
dosage for long periods of time, the practical superiority of medroxyprogesterone
for cancer therapy is evident.

The objective response of endometrial adenocarcinoma to medroxyprogesterone seems better related to the plasma levels than to the administered dose [26]. Indeed, high-dose medroxyprogesterone administration does not improve the objective remission rate [27]. The results of plasma level determinations are extremely controversial. As no direct dose–response relationship in the treatment of endometrial adenocarcinoma could be shown, medium-dose medroxyprogesterone administration, inducing plasma concentrations exceeding 90 ng/ml, achieves an excellent objective remission rate. We measured plasma concentrations easily exceeding the 90 ng/ml level after the first week of daily oral 150 mg Provera administration and after the fifth week of weekly intramuscular 1 g of Depo Provera. The progestational therapy should be continued for as long as the remission lasts; after discontinuing medroxyprogesterone treatment, striking relapses are often observed [13]. The responsiveness of the endometrial adenocarcinoma is directly related to the cytosol steroid receptor content of the tumour cells. The highest objective remission rates are achieved in patients bearing PR positive adenocarcinomas [8,10,28,29,30]. Moreover, the cytosol steroid receptor content of the endometrial adenocarcinoma directly determines both the hormone dependency and the degree of differentiation of the tumour. Finally, the steroid receptor content of the tumour is indirectly related to the metabolic and hormonal status of the host [31]: obesity, diabetes and oestrogenic milieu, as reflected by an initial oestrogenic vaginal smear, are important host factors favouring clinical response of the tumour [32]. As measurable tumour regression is to be expected, at the earliest, after 4–6 weeks' progestational therapy, monitoring of the responsiveness of the adenocarcinoma should be attempted. Hormone sensitivity to oral medroxyprogesterone treatment becomes apparent within 10 days by an abrupt fall of plasma LH levels, by an elevation of medroxyprogesterone plasma levels beyond 90 ng/ml, and by a sudden change toward atrophy in the vaginal smear. With intramuscular administration, the fall of plasma LH levels in the hormone-sensitive patients occurs as early as with oral administration, but it takes 5 weeks of treatment for the medroxyprogesterone plasma levels to attain a 90 ng/ml threshold and for the vaginal smear to become atrophic [33].

Medium-dose medroxyprogesterone treatment, even over a long period of time, does not cause significant side effects. Moreover, medroxyprogesterone very often procures the patient a sensation of well-being by relief of pain, improved appetite and gain in weight.

The hormonal approach to endometrial adenocarcinoma by means of anti-oestrogen therapy was initiated by the publication of one case report [34], and a 36% objective remission rate obtained following the administration of clomiphene citrate [35]. Later, tamoxifen at a daily dose of 20–40 mg was administered orally in first and second line treatment of metastatic or recurrent endometrial adenocarcinoma. A survey of approximately 50 patients with metastatic or recurrent endometrial adenocarcinoma treated by means of tamoxifen at conventional dosage, reveals an objective remission rate varying from 25%–57% lasting from 3 months up to more than 2 years [29,36,38,39,45].

Among the factors influencing the response of the endometrial adenocarcinoma to tamoxifen, the method of administration is practically of no account. Plasma concentrations ranging from 150–260 μg/ml are reached rapidly after regular daily administration of 20 mg tamoxifen. Finally, there is no evidence for a dose–response relationship for tamoxifen.

There is no proof that the responsiveness of the endometrial adenocarcinoma to tamoxifen is related to the cytosol oestrogen receptor content of the tumour cells. A close relationship is observed between the tumour responsiveness to medroxyprogesterone and to tamoxifen; the patients sensitive to second line tamoxifen therapy are those who previously responded to medroxyprogesterone [16,36]. While pulmonary metastases seem to respond to tamoxifen equally as well as vaginal recurrences, low-grade tumours with longer recurrence-free intervals are more likely to respond [36]. At the moment, tumour size is the only available parameter for monitoring the responsiveness of the endometrial adenocarcinoma to tamoxifen.

With conventional doses, possible side effects such as nausea or skin rashes, due to tamoxifen, are seldom observed and disappear after reducing the dose or stopping the treatment. Disturbing hot flushes are frequently experienced by younger patients.

Effects of Progestogens and Anti-oestrogens on Epithelial Ovarian Carcinomas

On an empirical basis, hormonal, especially anti-oestrogenic, therapy of epithelial ovarian carcinomas has been attempted. First, progestogens were introduced in the therapeutic scheme for ovarian cancer; more recently tamoxifen has been tried.

From the beginning of the 1970s until now, progestational treatment of ovarian cancer has been based on oral or intramuscular administration of high-dose medroxyprogesterone. The results on 183 patients have been published [40,41,42,43,44,45]. The remission rate of 0–15% is rather disappointing, taking into account the high cancericidal effect of medroxyprogesterone. The first results obtained in anti-oestrogenic second line treatment of advanced ovarian cancer by means of conventional tamoxifen administration are contradictory: the objective remission rate fluctuates between 8% and 100% [46,47].

Advances in hormone therapy of epithelial ovarian cancer could be made by selecting patients for first line treatment on account of the pathological characteristics (endometrioid and mesonephroid) and the cytosol steroid receptor content of the tumour, and by monitoring the treatment with medroxyprogesterone plasma level determinations.

Effects of Progestogens and Anti-oestrogens on Cervical and Vaginal Carcinomas

Endocervical adenocarcinoma represents only a small proportion of cervical carcinomas but the hormone responsiveness of this tumour has important therapeutic implications. It has been shown that adjuvant therapy with medium-

dose medroxyprogesterone following radiosurgical treatment of stage I endocervical adenocarcinoma reduces the recurrence rate [48]. Moreover, recurrent or
metastatic endocervical adenocarcinoma is as suitable for progestational therapy
as endometrial adenocarcinoma and even scores a higher objective remission rate
(70%) under medium-dose medroxyprogesterone administration [49].

As many cervical and some vaginal epitheliomas contain cytosol steroid
receptors, they can be considered as hormone responsive and treated with anti-
oestrogenic therapy. Even when steroid receptors are present in low concentrations or completely absent, the origin of the normal epithelium from the
Müllerian system justifies hormonal manipulation with tamoxifen–medroxyprogesterone combination therapy.

Conclusion

In the treatment of hormone-responsive gynaecological cancers, progestogens
and anti-oestrogens present different modes of action which seem complementary
to each other. Medroxyprogesterone attacks the hormone-dependent tumour cell
only by its anti-oestrogenic activity based on the simple mechanism of reducing
cytosol oestrogen receptor (ER) content. However, progestogens should finally
diminish their own efficiency by reduction of the cytosol PR without any stimulus
for their replacement. Tamoxifen on the other hand, attacks the cancer cell by a
more complex anti-oestrogenic action combined with the stimulation of PR
synthesis. Thus, for the future treatment of hormone-responsive cancers a possible synergism between the simple anti-oestrogenic action of medroxyprogesterone and the modulated and complex oestro—anti-oestrogenic activity of
tamoxifen could be established.

Hormonal therapy of a fully hormone-responsive ER+ PR+ cancer could be
started with medroxyprogesterone administration, which will transform the
tumour sooner or later to the slightly hormone-responsive ER+ PR− type by
consumption of the cytosol PR reserve. In the ER+ PR− tumour, tamoxifen
should attack the cancer cells by a combined oestro–anti-oestrogenic action,
depressing the cytosol ER content and inducing PR synthesis. In the hormone-
independent ER− PR− tumour, tamoxifen seems to act as an oestrogen, provok-
ing ER as well as PR synthesis, in that way priming the cancer for future
progestational therapy and transforming an autonomous cancer into a hormone-
dependent one.

While oral administration of tamoxifen at conventional dosage guarantees
efficient plasma concentrations, drug monitoring of therapy with medroxyprogesterone still remains problematic. Indeed, disagreement over the techniques of
plasma concentration measurement renders actual bio-availability of oral or
intramuscular, medium or high-dose medroxyprogesterone debatable.

References

1. Satyaswaroop PG, Frost A, Gurpide E (1980) Metabolism and effects of progesterone in the human endometrial adenocarcinoma cell line HEC-1. Steroids 35:21–37
2. Kimura J (1978) Effect of progesterone on cell division in chemically induced endometrial hyperplasia and adenocarcinoma in mice. Cancer Res 38:78–82
3. Ishiwata I, Udagawa H, Nozawa S (1978) Effects of progesterone on human endometrial carcinoma cells in vivo and in vitro. J Natl Cancer Inst 60:947–952
4. Barni S, Novelli GG, Zanoio L, Gerzeli G, Vecchietti G (1981) Chromatin analysis in human endometrial adenocarcinoma before and after treatment with MPA. Virchows Arch [Cell Pathol] 37:167–177
5. Vecchietti G, Gerzeli G, Zanoio L, Novelli GG, Barni S, Patton R (1981) Effetti del trattamento orale con 6-metil-17-idrossiprogesterone acetato (MAP) nell 'adenocarcinoma dell'endometrio. Minerva Ginecol 33:293–306
6. Vecchietti G, Gerzeli G, Zanoio L, Novelli GG, Barni S (1979). Effetti della terapia con medrossiprogesterone (MAP) sul contenuto in DNA dell 'adenocarcinoma dell'endometrio umano. Minerva Ginecol 31:597–603
7. Gurpide E, Tseng L, Gusberg SB (1977) Estrogen metabolism in normal and neoplastic endometrium. Am J Obstet Gynecol 129:809–816
8. Martin MP, Rolland PH, Gammerre M, Serment H, Toga M (1979) Estradiol and progesterone receptors in normal and neoplastic endometrium: correlations between receptors, histopathological examinations and clinical responses under progestin therapy. Int J Cancer 23:321–329
9. Vihko R, Jänne O, Kauppila A (1980) Steroid receptors in normal hyperplastic and malignant human endometria. Ann Clin Res 12:208–215
10. Gurpide E (1981) Hormone receptors in endometrial cancer. Cancer 48:638–641
11. Bonte J (1983) Traitement combiné par anti estrogènes et progestagènes en cancérologie gynécologique. Méd Hyg 41:1648–1661
12. Mortel R, Levy C, Wolff J-P, Nicolas J-C, Robel P, Baulieu E-E (1981) Female sex steroid receptors in postmenopausal endometrial carcinoma and biochemical response to an antiestrogen. Cancer Res 41:1140–1147
13. Bonte J, Drochmans A, Lassance M (1966) Traitement des adénocarcinomes du corps utérin par la médroxyprogestérone. Gyn Obstet (Paris) 65:179–185
14. Hustin J, Binard JM, Lambotte R (1976) Action des progestatifs de synthése sur le cancer endométrial. Critères cytochimiques. Ann Anat Pathol (Paris) 22:323–326
15. Ferenczy A (1977) Surface ultrastructural response of the human uterine lining epithelium to hormonal environment. A scanning electron microscopic study. Acta Cytol 21:566–572
16. Bonte J, Ide P, Billiet G, Wynants P (1981) Tamoxifen as a possible chemotherapeutic agent in endometrial adenocarcinoma. Gynecol Oncol 11:140–161
17. Groom GV, Griffiths K (1976) Effect of the anti-oestrogen tamoxifen on plasma levels of luteinizing hormone, follicle-stimulating hormone, prolactin, oestradiol and progesterone in normal pre-menopausal women. J Endocrinol 70:421–428
18. Ferrazzi E, Cartei G, Mattarazzo R, Fiorentino M (1977) Oestrogen-like effect of tamoxifen on vaginal epithelium (letter). Br Med J I:1351–1352
19. Bonte J, Kohorn I (1978) The response of hyperplastic, dysplastic and neoplastic endometrium to progestational therapy. In: Richardson GS, Maclaughlin DT (eds) Hormonal biology of endometrial cancer. UICC, Geneva, pp 155–184
20. Decoster JM, Bonte J, Marcq A (1977) Medroxyprogesterone acetate release from silastic devices as replacement for local irradiation by radium tubes in preoperative intrauterine packing for endometrial adenocarcinoma. Gynecol Oncol 5:189–195
21. Taylor RW (1981) The treatment of endometrial carcinoma with medroxyprogesterone acetate. In: Symposium on role of medroxyprogesterone acetate in endocrine-related tumors, Rome, 1981
22. Bokhman JV, Chepick OF, Volkova AT, Vishnevsky AS (1981). Adjuvant hormone therapy of primary endometrial carcinoma with oxyprogesterone caproate. Gynecol Oncol 11:371–378
23. von Fournier D, Kubli F, Bauer M, Weber E (1981) Hochdosierte Gestagen-Langzeittherapie beim Korpuskarzinom, Einfluss auf Uberlebenszeit. Geburtshilfe Frauenheilkd 41:266–269
24. Piver MS, Barlow JJ, Lurain JR, Blumenson LE (1980) Medroxyprogesterone acetate (Depo-Provera) versus hydroxyprogesterone caproate (Delalutin) in women with metastatic endometrial adenocarcinoma. Cancer 45:268–272

25. Caffier H, Horner G, Baum RJ (1982) Treatment of advanced or recurrent endometrial adeno-carcinoma with progestins, including medroxyprogesterone acetate. In: Proceedings of the international symposium on medroxyprogesterone acetate. Excerpta Medica, Geneva, pp 389–396

26. Pannutti F (1981) High doses of medroxyprogesterone acetate in advanced cancer treatment. Plasma levels and bioavailability after single and multiple dose administration. Preliminary results. In: Symposium on role of medroxyprogesterone acetate in endocrine-related tumors, Rome, 1981

27. Bernardo-Strada MR, Imparato E, Aspesi G, Pavesi L, Robustelli della Cuna G (1980) Il medrossiprogesterone acetato (MPA) ad alta dose per via orale nel trattamento delle fasi avanzate del cancro mammario ed endometriale. Minerva Med, 71:3241–3246

28. Benraad TJ, Friberg LG, Koenders AJM, Kullander S (1980) Do estrogen and progesterone receptors (E_2R and PR) in metastasizing endometrial cancers predict the response to gestogen therapy? Acta Obstet Gynecol Scand 59:155–159

29. Kauppila A, Fribert LG, (1981) Hormonal and cytotoxic chemotherapy for endometrial carcinoma. Acta Obstet Gynecol Scand [Suppl] 101:59–64

30. Ehrlich CE, Young PCM, Cleary RE (1981) Cytoplasmic progesterone and estradiol receptors in normal, hyperplastic, and carcinomatous endometria: Therapeutic implications. Am J Obstet Gynecol 141:539–546

31. Flickinger GL, Elsner C, Illingworth DV, Muechler EK, Mikhail G, (1977) Estrogen and progesterone receptors in the female genital tract of humans and monkeys. Ann NY Acad Sci 286:180–189

32. Bonte J, Drochmans A, Ide P, (1970) Cytologic evaluation of exclusive medroxyprogesterone acetate treatment for vaginal recurrence of endometrial adenocarcinoma. Acta Cytol 14:353–356

33. Bonte J (1979) Developments in endocrine therapy of endometrial and ovarian cancer. Rev Endocrin-Relat Cancer 3:11–17

34. Kistner RW (1966) Induction of ovulation with clomiphene citrate (Clomid). Obstet Gynecol Surv 20:873–900

35. Wall JA, Franklin RR, Kaufmann RH et al. (1965) The effects of clomiphene citrate on the endometrium. Am J Obstet Gynecol 93:842–849

36. Swenerton KD, Shaw D, White GW, Boyes DA (1979) Treatment of advanced endometrial carcinoma with tamoxifen. N Engl J Med 301:105

37. Broens J, Mouridsen HT, Serensen HM (1980) Tamoxifen in advanced endometrial carcinoma. Cancer Chemother Pharmacol 4:213

38. Hald I (1981) The use of tamoxifen ('Novadex') in endometrial cancer. Rev Endrocin-Relat Cancer [Suppl] 8:9–15

39. Quinn MA, Campbell JJ, Murray R, Pepperell RJ (1981) Tamoxifen and aminoglutethimide in the management of patients with advanced endometrial carcinoma not responsive to medroxy-progesterone. Aust NZ J Obstet Gynaecol 21:226–229

40. Malkasian GD Jr, Decker DG, Jorgensen EO, Edmonson JH (1977) Medroxyprogesterone acetate for the treatment of metastatic and recurrent ovarian carcinoma. Cancer Treat Rep 61:913–914

41. Mangioni C, Franceschi S, La Vecchia C, D'Incalci M (1981) High-dose medroxyprogesterone acetate (MPA) in advanced epithelial ovarian cancer resistant to first- or second-line chemotherapy. Gynecol Oncol 12:314–318

42. Slayton RE, Pagano M, Creech RH (1981) Progestin therapy for advanced ovarian cancer: A phase II Eastern Cooperative Oncology Group trial. Cancer Treat Rep 65:895–896

43 Aabo K, Pedersen AG, Hald I, Dombernowsky P (1982) High-dose medroxyprogesterone acetate (MPA) in advanced chemotherapy-resistant ovarian carcinoma: A phase II study. Cancer Treat 66:407–408

44. Mangioni C, Franceschi S, Landoni F, La Veccia C, Colombo E, Molina P (1982) High-dose progestin therapy for advanced ovarian cancer. An updated report. In: Proceedings of the international symposium on medroxyprogesterone acetate. Excerpta Medica, Geneva, pp 461–467

45. Trope C, Johnson JE, Sigurdsson K, Simonsen E (1982) High-dose medroxyprogesterone acetate for the treatment of advanced ovarian carcinoma. Cancer Treat Rep 66:1441-1443

46. Myers AM, Moore GE, Major FJ (1981) Advanced ovarian carcinoma: Response to antiestrogen therapy. Cancer 48:2368–2370

47. Schwartz PE, Keating G, MacLusky N, Naftolin F, Eisenfeld A (1982) Tamoxifen therapy for advanced ovarian cancer. Obstet Gynecol 59:583–588

48. Bonte J (1975) Récents progrèse dans l'hormonoprophylaxie et l'hormonothérapie de l'adénocarcinome utérin par médroxyprogestérone. Med Hyg 33:1831–1833

49. Bonte J, Decoster JM, Ide P, Billiet G, (1978) Hormonoprophylaxis and hormonotherapy in the treatment of endometrial adneocarcinoma by means of medroxyprogesterone acetate. Gynecol Oncol 6:60–75

13 · Epidemiology of Endometrial Cancer

M.P. Vessey and M. Lawless

Vital Statistical Data

An examination of the available vital statistical data on incidence and mortality is a good starting point for a review of the epidemiology of any disease. Unfortunately, this task is unusually difficult for endometrial cancer for a number of reasons. (Although not strictly correct, the terms 'endometrial cancer' and 'corpus cancer' are used interchangeably in this article.) First, it is not always easy for the histopathologist to distinguish atypical endometrial hyperplasia from endometrial cancer—doubts about where to draw the line could obviously have an important influence on incidence rates. Secondly, death certificates (and to a lesser extent cancer registrations) are sometimes so poorly completed that it is not indicated whether the cancer arose in the cervix or in the body of the uterus. These cases have to be put in a 'site not specified' category and, although there is some evidence that the majority are corpus cancers [1], they have greatly complicated the interpretation of time trends. Thirdly, the correct denominator for computing incidence or mortality rates is obviously the population of women with intact uteri. This figure, however, is often unknown so that the total population is generally used. This results in an underestimation of the risk for those who have not undergone hysterectomy and, more importantly, further difficulty in assessing secular trends. These problems should be borne in mind in evaluating what follows.

Table 13.1 gives the incidence rates for cancer of the body of the uterus from the Birmingham and West Midlands Regional Cancer Registry for the years 1968–1976. It can be seen that although the rates fluctuate from year to year, there is little sign of a trend over this period in any age group. Figure 13.1 shows that the mortality rates for England and Wales during the interval 1968–1980 slowly declined at ages below 65 years. In computing these figures, we included deaths

Table 13.1. Age-specific incidence rates per 100 000 for cancer of the body of the uterus (ICD 182.0) for the years 1968–1976. Data from the Birmingham and West Midlands Cancer Registry, England

Age group (years)	Year								
	1968	1969	1970	1971	1972	1973	1974	1975	1976
40–44	4	8	4	7	5	5	5	3	4
45–49	19	13	11	16	10	13	13	13	18
50–54	33	27	28	31	29	27	26	39	36
55–59	39	32	30	30	33	44	38	42	39
60–64	42	32	43	43	39	49	47	49	47
65–69	47	44	51	46	43	49	51	41	55
70–74	39	48	52	45	38	41	36	41	43

coded to the 'site not specified' category as well as those coded to carcinoma of the corpus. It should be noted, however, that the 'site not specified' category formed a small and fairly constant proportion of the total over the whole period and that the general pattern of mortality is much the same (although, of course, with rates at a generally lower level) for carcinoma of the corpus alone.

Vital statistical data for the United States show entirely different patterns from those for England and Wales. First, most cancer registries noted a marked increase in incidence rates during the late 1960s and early 1970s, especially among women in the years immediately following the menopause [2]. This is illustrated by data reported by Walker and Jick [3] collected by the Commission on Professional and Hospital Activities—Professional Activity Study (Fig.13.2). Subsequently, the elevated rates in this age group (though not in others) declined. This phenomenon has been related to the rise and fall in the sales of conjugated equine oestrogens for 'hormone replacement therapy'. Secondly, a high (but steadily declining) proportion of uterine cancer deaths in the United States are in the 'site not specified' category. As can be seen from Figs. 13.3–13.5, exclusion of the 'site not specified' cancers leads to the conclusion that endometrial cancer death rates are rising, while their inclusion (which is likely to give the more accurate picture) leads to the conclusion that endometrial cancer death rates are falling!

Looking at the incidence of corpus cancer on a wider international basis, rates tend to be high in the affluent industrialised countries and low in the less industrialised developing countries. This is shown in Fig. 13.6, which also illustrates the fact that, as is the case with breast cancer, corpus cancer incidence in different countries is closely correlated with per caput total fat consumption [4].

Risk Factors

Risk factors for endometrial cancer have been assessed in a large number of epidemiological studies, mostly of case-control design. During the past decade,

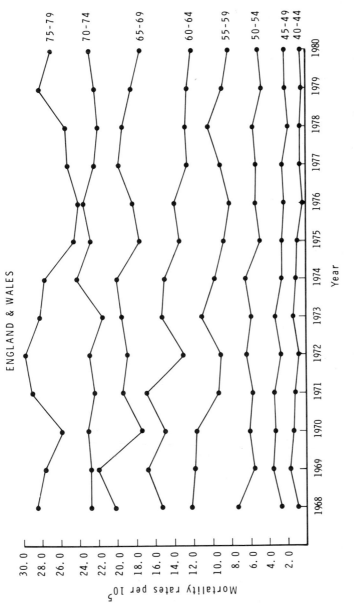

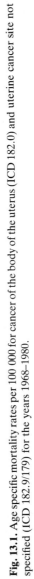

Fig. 13.1. Age specific mortality rates per 100 000 for cancer of the body of the uterus (ICD 182.0) and uterine cancer site not specified (ICD 182.9/179) for the years 1968–1980.

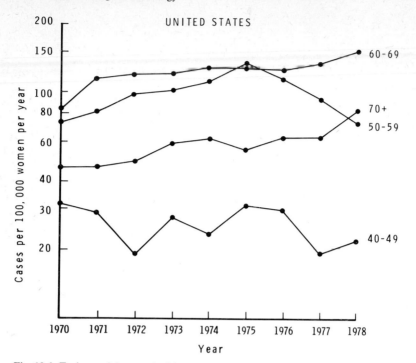

Fig. 13.2. Endometrial cancer incidence rates per 100 000 for women with an intact uterus for the years 1970–1978. Note that the vertical scale is logarithmic. (Walker and Jick [3])

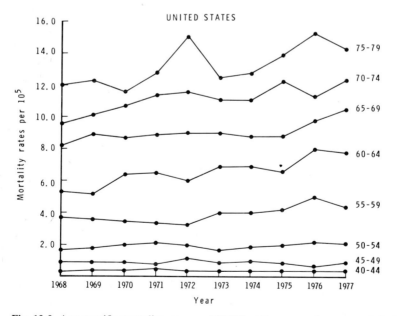

Fig. 13.3. Age-specific mortality rates per 100 000 white women for cancer of the body of the uterus (ICD 182.0) for the years 1968–1977.

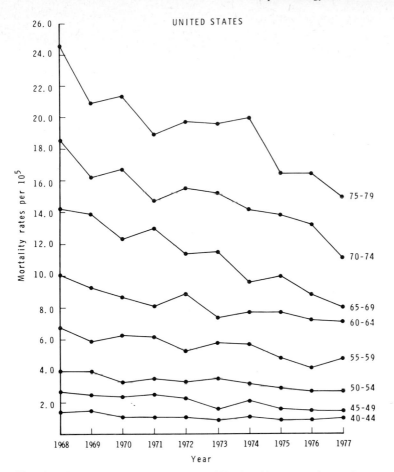

Fig. 13.4. Age-specific mortality rates per 100 000 white women for uterine cancer site not specified (ICD 182.9) for the years 1968–1977.

the great majority of such studies have primarily been concerned with the relationship between hormone replacement therapy (or oral contraceptive use) and endometrial cancer, but many of these investigations have also provided information about other relevant factors. Table 13.2 summarises the risk factors which have been found reasonably consistently in clinical and epidemiological studies. They are well known, so that no general review is necessary, but it is worth noting that most of them can be reconciled on the basis of the 'oestrogen excess' hypothesis [5]. In particular, the association with obesity is probably explicable in terms of the peripheral conversion of androstenedione to oestrone in adipose tissue (with the subsequent conversion of oestrone to oestradiol) while it is possible that the associations with diabetes and hypertension are due at least in part to the tendency for these conditions to occur in those who are overweight.

Table 13.2. Risk factors for endometrial cancer

Factor	High risk	Low risk	Approximate magnitude of relative risk, high risk to low risk		
			>4	2–4	<2
Age	Old	Young	*		
Parity	Nulliparous	Parous		*	
Age at menarche	Early	Late			*
Age at menopause	Late	Early			*
Body build	Obese	Thin	*		
Diabetes	Present	Absent		*	
Hypertension	Present	Absent			*
Stein–Leventhal syndrome	Present	Absent		?	
Oestrogen secreting ovarian tumours	Present	Absent		?	
Previous breast cancer	Present	Absent			*
Previous ovarian cancer	Present	Absent			*
Oestrogen therapy	Present	Absent	*		
Sequential oral contraceptive therapy	Present	Absent		*	
Radiation exposure	Present	Absent		*	

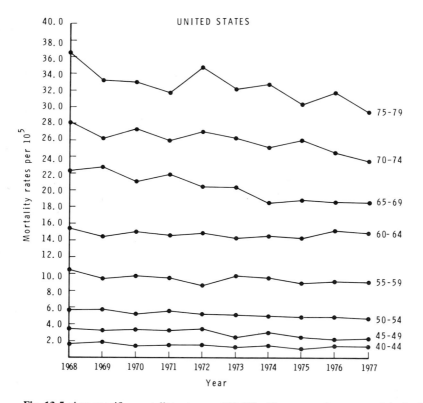

Fig. 13.5. Age-specific mortality rates per 100 000 white women for cancer of the body of the uterus (ICD 182.0) and uterine cancer site not specified (ICD 182.9) for the years 1968–1977.

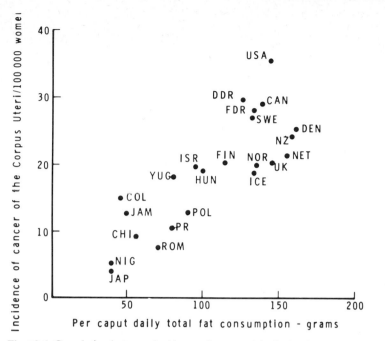

Fig. 13.6. Correlation between incidence of cancer of the body of the uterus and per caput daily total fat consumption in 23 countries. (Armstrong and Doll [4])

From the point of view of preventing endometrial cancer, the strong influences of obesity and oestrogen replacement therapy deserve special consideration. Most papers do not provide sufficient information about the distribution of body weight in cases and controls to allow the effect of this factor to be explored in detail, but Table 13.3 shows data from an early report by Wynder et al. [6] and Table 13.4 from a very recent one by Henderson et al. [7]. It can be seen that both

Table 13.3. Weight of women with endometrial cancer and of control subjects at ages 50–59 years. Data modified from Wynder et al. [6]

Weight[a]	% women with endometrial cancer (n = 90)	% control women (n = 150)	Relative risks, cases: controls
Below average weight by			
21 lb or more	7	12	0.9
10–20 lb	9	20	0.7
3–9 lb	10	19	0.9
Average weight ± 2 lb	8	13	1.0
Above average weight by			
3–9 lb	9	9	1.6
10–20 lb	11	9	2.0
21–50 lb	28	15	3.1
51 lb or more	18	3	9.8

[a] Height and age-specific weight tables were used to classify each patient's deviation from average weight.

Table 13.4. Weight of women 1 year prior to diagnosis of endometrial cancer and of control subjects. Data modified from Henderson et al. [7][a]

Weight	% women with endometrial cancer ($n = 110$)	% control women ($n = 110$)	Relative risk, cases: controls
Up to 129 lb	25	46	1.0
130–149 lb	25	35	1.4
150–169 lb	10	9	2.0
170–189 lb	12	5	9.6
190 lb or more	28	5	17.7

[a] All women in this study were aged 45 years or less. Closely similar results were obtained when the data were classified by Quetelet's index (weight/height^2).

these papers indicate an extremely high risk in excessively heavy women. Data on the risks associated with oestrogen replacement therapy are extensive and have been reviewed on many occasions [8–10]. It must suffice to note here (a) that cancers induced by oestrogen replacement therapy usually seem to be detected at a relatively early stage (perhaps as a result of surveillance of women receiving treatment) and are often of a favourable histological grade, with an accordingly good prognosis, (b) that the cancer risk increases with duration of use and dose of oestrogen and appears to decline fairly soon after cessation of therapy, and (c) that there is considerable, although not conclusive, evidence that the addition of a progestogen to the oestrogen will eliminate the cancer risk.

Oral Contraceptives

An important recent advance in our knowledge of the epidemiology of endometrial cancer is the discovery that combined oral contraceptives seem to protect against the disease. The earliest data to suggest this were published by Weiss and Sayvetz in 1980 [11]. These workers, in a case-control study including 117 women aged 35–54 years with endometrial cancer and 395 healthy women, found the sequential oral contraceptive, Oracon, to increase the risk of endometrial cancer sevenfold and combined oral contraceptives to reduce the risk by 50%. As Table 13.5 shows, six other case-control studies published since then have produced similar results [7,12–16]. All of these studies, however, are on the small side while two [13,15] include many older women who could not have been exposed to the pill. Accordingly, there is a need for more extensive data to clarify the precise nature of the protective effect of the pill, and this is likely to be derived from the study being conducted by the Centers for Disease Control which should eventually include several hundred cases. In the meantime, there is evidence that the protective effect increases with duration of use and that it persists, at least for some years, after discontinuation of use (Table 13.6). Some authors have found that the protective effect is more prominent with the strongly progestogenic pills and that use of menopausal oestrogen therapy can eliminate the benefit. Henderson et al. [7] found clear evidence of reduced risk only in women who had had less than three live births and who weighed less than 170 lb.

Table 13.5. Case-control studies of oral contraceptive use and endometrial cancer

| First author [Ref.] | Country | Endometrial cancer cases | | Relative risk: ever-use to never-use combined pills[a] |
		Age range	Number	
Weiss [11]	USA	35–54	117	0.5 (0.1–1.0)
Kaufman [12]	USA	–59	154	0.5 (0.3–0.8)
Kelsey [13]	USA	45–74	167	0.6
Hulka [14]	USA	–59	79	0.4
La Vecchia [15]	Italy	–84	173	0/173 cases and 12/347 controls exposed
CDC [16]	USA	20–54	187	0.5 (0.3–0.8)
Henderson [7]	USA	–45	127	0.5

[a] Figures in parentheses indicate 95% confidence limits (not always given by author). CDC = centers for disease control

Table 13.6. Case-control studies of oral contraceptive use and endometrial cancer. Data on duration of use and recency of use of combined pills

First author [ref.]	Increasing protection with duration of use?	Persistent protection after stopping use?
Weiss [11]	Not after 1 year's use	For a year or two
Kaufman [12]	Yes	For at least 5 years
Kelsey [13]	Yes	Not stated
Hulka [14]	Yes	Effect wanes
La Vecchia [15]	No data	No data
CDC [16]	Not after 1 year's use	For at least 10 years
Henderson [17]	Yes	Not stated

The major cohort studies concerned with the long term effects of oral contraceptive use still include too few cases of endometrial cancer for conclusions to be drawn. It may be noted, however, that such data as are available are in support of the findings in the case control studies [17,18].

Comment

In contrast to breast cancer, for which preventive medicine has little to offer at present, there seem to be grounds for optimism that many cases of endometrial cancer might be avoided by control of body weight, avoidance of unopposed oestrogen therapy, and use of combined oral contraceptives. The last mentioned measure is particularly important because combined oral contraceptives are being used on an ever-increasing scale. If it is clearly shown that the protective effect persists for 20 years or more after discontinuation, a substantial decline in the incidence of endometrial cancer may occur in developed countries in the next decade or so.

References

1. Weiss NS (1978) Assessing the risks from menopausal estrogen use: What can we learn from trends in mortality from uterine cancer. J Chron Dis 31:705–708
2. Weiss NS, Szekely DR, Austin DF (1976) Increasing incidence of endometrial cancer in the United States. New Engl J Med 294:1259–1262
3. Walker AM, Jick H (1980) Declining rates of endometrial cancer. Obstet Gynecol 56:733–736
4. Armstrong BK, Doll R (1975) Environmental factors and cancer incidence and mortality in different countries with special reference to dietary practices. Int J Cancer. 15:617–631
5. Henderson BE, Ross RK, Pike MC, Casagrande JT (1982) Endogenous hormones as a major factor in human cancer. Cancer Res. 42:3232–3239
6. Wynder EL, Escher GC, Mantel N (1966) An epidemiological investigation of cancer of the endometrium. Cancer 19:489–520
7. Henderson BE, Casagrande JT, Pike MC, Mack T, Rosario I, Duke A (1983) The epidemiology of endometrial cancer in young women. Br J Cancer 47:749–756
8. Mack TM (1978) Uterine cancer and estrogen therapy. Front Hormone Res. 5:101–116
9. Smith PG, Vessey MP (1981) Oestrogen use and endometrial cancer—epidemiological aspects. In: Jordan JA, Singer A (Eds) Controversies in gynaecological oncology. Royal College of Obstetricians and Gynaecologists, London, pp 81–90
10. British Gynaecological Cancer Group (1981) Oestrogen replacement therapy and endometrial cancer. Lancet I:1359–1360
11. Weiss NS, Sayvetz TA (1980) Incidence of endometrial cancer in relation to the use of oral contraceptives. New Engl J Med 302:551–554
12. Kaufman DW, Shapiro S, Slone D, Rosenberg L, Miettinen OS, Stolley PD (1980) Decreased risk of endometrial cancer among oral contraceptive users. New Engl J Med 303:1045:1047
13. Kelsey JL, Li Volsi VA, Holford TR, Fischer DB, Mostow ED, Schwartz PE (1982) A case-control study of cancer of the endometrium. Am J Epidemiol 116:333–342
14. Hulka BS, Chambless LE, Kaufman DG, Fowler WC, Greenberg BG (1982) Protection against endometrial carcinoma by combination-product oral contraceptives. JAMA 247:475–477
15. La Vecchia C, Franceschi S, Gallus G, Decarli A, Colombo E, Mangioni C (1982) Oestrogens and obesity as risk factors for endometrial cancer in Italy. Int J Epidemiol ll:120–126
16. Centers for Disease Control Cancer and Steroid Hormones Study (1983) Oral contraceptive use and the risk of endometrial cancer. JAMA 249:1600–1604
17. Kay CR (1980) Progestogens before and after the menopause. Br Med J 281:811–812
18. Ramcharan S, Pellegrin FA, Ray R, Hsu J-P (1981) The Walnut Creek Contraceptive Drug Study. A prospective study of the side effects of oral contraceptives. Volume III. National Institutes of Health, Bethesda, MD

Acknowledgements. We are grateful to Dr. J. Waterhouse for providing the information about cancer of the body of the uterus from the Birmingham and West Midlands Regional Cancer Registry and to Mrs. D. Collinge for secretarial assistance.

14 · The Place for Radiotherapy in Endometrial Cancer

C.A. Joslin

Introduction

The incidence of cancer of the endometrium is increasing and in the United Kingdom almost equals that of cervical cancer. Clinically, it most commonly presents as stage I disease, being locally confined to the endometrial and myometrial tissues. However, depending upon the grade of tumour and depth of myometrial invasion the chance of regional spread to the pelvic lymph nodes can be as high as 50% [1]. Management for stage I endometrial cancer is therefore not only concerned with the eradication of disease in the primary organ, but also with determining the likelihood of pelvic node involvement and providing appropriate treatment.

Disease extension into the isthmus and endocervical regions (stage II) has a greater chance of regional spread with a worse prognosis. Fortunately, such spread generally occurs late in the natural history of the disease and does not constitute a common presentation and will not be specifically dealt with in this presentation.

On an historical note in 1922 Regaud [2] found that the adenomatous structures of the bull's testis are extremely radioresistant. Unfortunately these findings were applied to adenomatous tissues in general, including the endometrium. This gave support to the view, commonly held at that time, that radium was for the cervix and surgery for the corpus. Despite such opinion Heyman [3] achieved remarkable success when using radium alone for treating endometrial cancer, and by systematically using a uterine packing system the Radiumhemmett reported excellent results for stage I disease. In view of this it is first necessary to address the problem of whether radiotherapy offers an effective alternative to surgery alone.

Radiotherapy Alone or Surgery Alone

The best evidence is from Stockholm where Kottmeier [4] reported a 5-year recovery rate of 76% for a series of 369 clinically operable patients. However, treatment failed in 66 patients who were then salvaged by surgery and the true radium cure rate was 63%, which corresponds to the level of results reported by others. Such results for radiotherapy above are inferior to those for surgery alone, which average 75% [5], irrespective of whether an abdominal hysterectomy and bilateral salpingo-oophorectomy (BSO) or Wertheim hysterectomy is used. Thus, it becomes difficult to make the case for intracavitary radiotherapy as the sole means of treatment. Indeed Kottmeier moved to a situation where routine hysterectomy was done in those patients considered as good surgical risks 6 weeks after an exposure of 1.55 C kg^{-1} (6000 roentgens) at a myometrial depth of 1 cm given by two or three packings with Heyman's capsules at intervals of 2–4 weeks.

While the case for surgery is fairly well established for the clinically operable patient, there are also patients who are technically operable although not clinically suitable. Such patients are often fit enough for intracavitary treatment and it is therefore necessary to consider the best type of intracavitary treatment to use.

Intracavitary Dosimetry

Several types of intracavitary treatment are available, each offering some form of advantage and having some disadvantage. When considering the various methods it is important that the natural behaviour of the spread of disease is taken into account. Generally, the pattern of disease spread is along the surface of the endometrium, and also invading the myometrium as far as the serosal covering. The majority of lesions arise within the uterine fundus and it is, therefore, important to choose a treatment method which will provide an isodose envelope which is wider at the fundus than in the region of the endocervix. It is also important that the rate of fall-off in dose from the intrauterine sources is sufficiently restricted still to allow a cancerocidal dose to be delivered at the fundal serosa. This becomes particularly difficult to ensure when using a single line source technique such as the Manchester system. One alternative is the Heyman technique which offers two major advantages: (1) by tightly packing the uterine cavity with source capsules the uterine wall can be stretched and a closer approximation of the sources to the tumour obtained, and (2) the system delivers a more evenly distributed dose to the myometrial tissues.

Afterloading

A major problem with the preloaded treatment systems and particularly the Heyman system is that of exposure of staff to irradiation. Generally, the same problems exist as for cancer of the cervix and they can be overcome by using various forms of afterloading. However, for practical reasons most of these systems use a single line source and, by changing the source loadings, can be used for treating either cervical or corpus cancer.

Of the afterloaded systems designed specifically for treating endometrial cancer one, introduced by Strickland in 1965 [6], uses a helix of stainless steel wire to form a loop in the uterine cavity. It is loaded manually with individual 240.5 MBq (6.5 mCi) sources of cobalt-60 to a total loading of 2.22–2.59 GBq (60–75 mCi). When compared with a single line source the device offers an improved dose distribution and reduces staff exposure to about 0.25 mSv (25 mrem) for each loading. A dose of 60 Gy (6000 rad) at a distance of 1.5 cm from the helix is delivered in two fractions of 15 h each, spaced a week apart. Using this technique alone a 5-year disease-free rate of 60% is claimed.

Simon and Silverstone [7] have produced a method of converting the Heyman's system to afterloading. Each capsule is afterloaded with 925 MBq (25 mCi) of caesium-137 carried on a stainless steel wire. Using this system the staff exposure is reduced to only 10 or 20 mSv (1 or 2 mrem).

Combined External and Intracavitary Therapy

The argument for combining external beam and intracavitary therapy arises because of the high chance of pelvic node involvement, particularly in those cases having myometrial invasion. The effect of the external beam therapy is to provide a cancerocidal effect on the pelvic lymph nodes.

The early results reported for this treatment method were extremely poor. Randall and Goddard in 1956 [8] reported on 76 patients treated by a combination of radium and orthovoltage therapy having a 24% 5-year survival. Lampe in 1963 [9] reported 5-year survival rates of 58% for stage I and 24% for stage II disease using a combination of teletherapy and radium. There are many who now treat stage II patients with a course of external teletherapy to a pelvic dose of 40–45 Gy (4000–4500 rad) in 20 fractions over 28 days, followed 1–2 weeks later by some form of intracavitary treatment. However, the publications are sparse when it comes to reporting results and the numbers are small, but claims for survival rates of up to 50% or more are made.

In support of using external beam therapy there is evidence to show that it does exert some influence on the primary tumour. Delclos and Fletcher [10] have reported control of pelvic disease in 45% of unresectable cases receiving less than 30 Gy (3000 rad) and 77% in patients receiving more than this; most would now give 40–50 Gy in 4–5 weeks.

In fairness, the results for combined intracavitary and external beam therapy should be contrasted with radical regional surgery such as a Wertheim hysterectomy. Wertheim hysterectomy was advocated by Lewis [11] and Javert [12], whereas Lees [13] and Shah and Green [14] did not, since the rates of recurrence were not affected. Lewis later advocated postoperative radiotherapy following Wertheim hysterectomy [15].

Di Saia and Creasman advocate a non-radical surgical approach in well differentiated stage I lesions, provided that there is only superficial disease present limited to the uterus [16].

In summary, the use of surgery alone for stage I endometrial cancer as opposed to radiotherapy alone still has the support of the majority of clinicians. A clinical trial would put this to the test, but with 5-year cure rates of 81% reported in a review by Salazar [17] for surgery alone, it would be difficult to make a convincing case for such a study.

Preoperative Intracavitary or Postoperative Intravaginal Irradiation as an Adjunct to Surgery

While it is generally considered that surgery combined with some form of intracavitary radiation provides results which are superior to surgery alone, the review by Jones [5] suggests that the results are no different. However, this evaluation was unable to assess the grading of tumours, and patients receiving joint therapy may have been those with higher grade tumours. Support for Jones' conclusions comes from Graham [18], who carried out a random trial of hysterectomy versus preoperative intracavitary radium versus postoperative intravaginal radium. The results were: surgery alone 64%, preoperative radium 76%, postoperative radium 81%. The differences are not significant at the $P = 0.05$ level.

Piver in 1980 [19] reported a prospective study comparing hysterectomy alone, preoperative uterine radium and postoperative vaginal radium in 189 stage I cancers. All patients were followed for 10 years with an overall survival rate of 93% for the combined groups. For grade I lesions survival was 94.0%, grade II 94% and grade III 70.0%. Survival for the different treatments was 96% for postoperative, 93% for preoperative radiotherapy and for surgery alone 90%. An important finding was the rate of vaginal vault recurrence, which occurred in 7.5% having surgery only, 4.5% of the preoperative radiotherapy group and 0% in the postoperative radiotherapy group.

Preoperative Intracavitary Radiation

The results from Kuipers [20], in a review on behalf of the European Curietherapy Group of 604 patients treated by various preoperative intracavitary techniques, gave a 5-year survival rate of 75% for stage I disease. This seems to support the views of Jones, Piver and Graham in terms of survival, and thus the possible value of preoperative intracavitary therapy needs further consideration. Among the advantages claimed is a reduction in vaginal vault metastases resulting from operative spillage or lymphatic permeation. On these grounds alone many support the view that preoperative radiation should be given routinely.

Another advantage claimed is that it shrinks the primary tumour, making surgery easier. Certainly a number of reports have shown that this group have little residual tumour following irradiation. Some have attempted to relate the intracavitary dose to residual disease and to survival. Boronow [21] reported using 4000 to 4500 milligram hours preoperatively in 714 cases with an 85% 5-year survival, and 96% 5-year survival when using between 5000 to 5500 milligram hours: however, this trend was not supported for yet higher doses. Dally [22] reported a 5-year survival of 54% for one preoperative intracavitary insertion and 66% for two insertions. Unfortunately such results, and this applies to the vast majority of reports for surgery with or without preoperative irradiation, were given little or no critical evaluation regarding any possible imbalance of tumour grading or depth of myometrial involvement which might prejudice survival. One exception is the study by Salazar [17] who showed that combined therapy reduces the pelvic failure rate in grade III tumours.

On review of the literature there appears to be a consensus of opinion that preoperative intracavitary radiation reduces the chance of local, lymphatic, and vascular dissemination of cancer at hysterectomy: however, there is little evidence to support these views apart from a reduction in vaginal vault recurrences. The disadvantages, as pointed out by Strickland, include a possible delay of definitive surgery by several weeks. It distorts the histopathological picture of the tumour and makes any estimation of myometrial invasion difficult. The morbidity reported varies but cannot be ignored. Boronow [21] reported a 16% complication rate in 90 patients treated preoperatively with Heyman's capsules and vaginal ovoids followed by surgery.

Postoperative Intravaginal Therapy

One alternative to preoperative intracavitary treatment is that of postoperative intravaginal therapy. A number of reports have been produced giving a 5-year survival rate equal to, or better than, preoperative intracavitary radiation; however, as already discussed, no one has shown this trend to be significant.

Kuipers [20] reported an 85% 5-year survival for postoperative radiotherapy but for many cases this included external beam therapy.

A reduction in vaginal vault recurrence matching those for preoperative intracavitary treatment has been claimed, and this is its major advantage. Even when this treatment is refined by using a vaginal obturator to fit the full length of the vagina, such as that described by Dobbie [23], survival rates are no better.

The most obvious case for radiotherapy given either as preoperative intracavitary or postoperative intravaginal therapy is that it reduces the incidence of vaginal vault recurrence (Table 14.1). Some, however, would argue that a larger vaginal cuff removed at surgery would do likewise. Against this is the fact that it

Table 14.1. Vaginal vault recurrence rates

Reference	Surgery alone (%)	Preoperative intracavitary (%)	Postoperative intravaginal (%)
Piver [19]	7.5	4.5	0
Joslin [28]	Not studied	–	<1.5
Purcell and Underwood [29]	18.4	Not reported	Not reported
Graham [18]	12.0	3	0
Dobbie [30]	5.5	0	1.8
Rutledge, Tan and Fletcher [31]	20.0	1.5	–
Beiler, Schmutz and O'Rourke [32]	12.0	1.6	

would not eliminate suburethral or lower vaginal recurrence as postoperative intravaginal treatments can do, provided a suitable obturator is used to treat the lower vagina. Nevertheless, there is morbidity resulting from such treatment, particularly vaginal stenosis and also proctitis.

The Place for External Beam Therapy

The lack of difference in survival rates for either radical hysterectomy alone or combined with pre- or postoperative intracavitary therapy can be shown to relate to the fact that in many patients disease has spread to involve the pelvic nodes. In particular, the grade of tumour and ensuing spread of disease to involve the pelvic lymph nodes and para-aortic nodes is important (Table 14.2). Also, the chance of pelvic lymph node involvement is related to the depth of myometrial invasion as well as to tumour grade (Table 14.2) and these two prognostic factors are inter-related (Table 14.3). Thus, if we are to provide an increased chance of cure for patients with grade III tumours or deep myometrial invasion, we need to do more than remove the primary organ and treat the vaginal tissues. If surgery alone is to achieve this it must be equivalent to a Wertheim hysterectomy. However, as already discussed it appears to be no better than routine total hysterectomy and bilateral salpingo-oophorectomy (BSO). In view of this the role of external beam therapy needs consideration.

External beam therapy has been used both preoperatively with or without intracavitary therapy and postoperatively with or without intravaginal therapy.

Preoperative External Beam Therapy

Lampe used deep X-ray therapy to deliver 40-Gy (4000 rad) in 3–4 weeks in 121 patients with stage I disease followed by a hysterectomy and BSO 6 weeks later. He reported a 90% 5-year survival compared with another group of 52 patients treated by surgery and postoperative intravaginal therapy, which gave a 69% 5-year survival [9].

Table 14.2. Incidence of pelvic node involvement for stage I Ca corpus

Reference	Myometrial invasion (%)	
	Superficial	Deep
Javert [12]	6.2	50
Liu and Meigs [33]	4.0	45
Delclos and Fletcher [10]	7.0	18
Lewis [15]	0	36
Creasman et al. [27]	11.5	43

	Tumour grade		
	G1	G2	G3
Lewis, Stallworthy and Cowdell [11]	5.5	10	26
Creasman et al. [27]	3.0	10	36
(Para-aortic rate)	(1.5)	(4.0)	(28)

Table 14.3. Relationship between degree of differentiation and depth of myometrial invasion

| | | Histology | | |
| | No. of | Well | Moderately or poorly | Not |
Infiltration	cases	differentiated	differentiated	known
Superficial	67	63	2	
Less than half myometrial thickness	82	69	12	
More than half myometrial thickness	107	78	27	
Total	256	210	41	5
Recurrences over 5 years	25	16	9	–

Ritcher et al. [24] reported a 95% 5-year survival in 161 patients with stage I disease, the majority of whom had preoperative external beam radiotherapy. The dose delivered ranged from 10.5 to 67 Gy at a rate of 1.8–2.0 Gy per day, most patients receiving 35 Gy. This was followed one to two weeks later by surgery, and very few complications were encountered.

Gagnon [25] reported on 24 stage II patients receiving preoperative external beam therapy. A dose of 45–50 Gy was given. Surgery 4–5 weeks later in 23 of these patients revealed local residual disease in 14 of them (61%), suggesting, for the dose given, that external beam therapy alone will not cure extensive local disease. The adjusted survival rate at 5 years was estimated at 81%. Of the four recurrences by 5 years one was vaginal, one had pulmonary metastases, one liver metastases and one abdominal metastases.

Salazar et al. [17] reported on preoperative therapy according to uterine size. For a small uterus, a tandem and ovoids were used to deliver 30 Gy to the Manchester point A, followed by 50 Gy to the central pelvis and 45 Gy to the pelvic side wall with supervoltage therapy. For a large uterus, Heyman's capsules were used to deliver 40 Gy at 1 cm into the myometrium and external therapy as before.

Of the 155 cases only four (2.5%) failed in the pelvis. Surgical complications occurred in 10% and there were 5% chronic radiation problems. 82% were alive at 5 years without evidence of disease. On reviewing the literature Salazar reported 87% survival in 362 cases. This is significantly better ($P<0.05$) than that of patients treated with initial surgery (80%) or preoperative intracavitary therapy (80%). Also, the recurrence rates appeared lower in the preoperative external beam therapy group than in any other group.

Postoperative External Beam Therapy

One of the very few prospective randomised trials carried out to assess postoperative external pelvic irradiation in stage I disease is by Onsrud [26]. He compared postoperative intravaginal radiotherapy with or without external radiotherapy in 386 patients. Intravaginal therapy was used to deliver 60 Gy to the vaginal vault. Patients were then randomised to receive or not receive external radiotherapy of 40 Gy to the whole pelvis. The survival rates were the same: however, the number of vaginal and pelvic recurrences was higher in patients not receiving external radiotherapy. Unfortunately for the study those receiving external radiotherapy had a higher number of distant metastases. Creasman et al. [27] showed that the number of aortic nodes involved can be quite high (28%) compared with 36% pelvic node involvement. External therapy to the pelvis alone would therefore fail to treat one area at risk, which may help to account for Onsrud's results.

Joslin has reported using postoperative intravaginal and external beam therapy [28]. Intravaginal therapy is given using a Perspex obturator loaded to treat the vagina down to the suburethral region. The obturator is afterloaded using a high-activity afterloading device, delivering dose rates of the order of 5 Gy min^{-1} at 0.5 cm from the obturator surface. When used without external beam therapy a total dose of 35 Gy in 5 fractions at a depth of 0.5 cm from the obturator surface was given in 4 days, later reduced to 30 Gy in 5 fractions. Initially, this technique was used for all stage I cases with no external therapy. However, it soon became clear that pelvic recurrence rates and survival were adversely affected as the depth of myometrial invasion increased. As a result, external beam therapy was added and the intravaginal dose reduced. A prescribed tumour dose of 35 Gy delivered in 15 fractions over 21 days followed by intravaginal treatment of 20 Gy in 4 fractions over 3 days was given. The latter has since been reduced to 16 Gy in 4 fractions for a 3 cm diameter obturator and 12 Gy in 4 fractions for smaller obturators.

The results indicate that patients receiving external beam therapy fare better than those who receive intravaginal therapy only. In particular, a reduction in pelvic recurrences occurred, particularly for the deeply invasive group, as a result of adding external beam therapy ($P \leq 0.01$). However, this improvement was not maintained for less invasive disease. In terms of survival this pattern was reversed due to the deeply invasive group developing metastases outside the pelvis, and the significance of myometrial invasion as a prognostic indicator is extremely high despite such cases having external beam therapy.

Recurrence in relation to histological grading was assessed in 251 patients. Of these, 210 had well differentiated tumours of which 4 spread to distant sites, and 41 patients had poorly differentiated tumours of which 5 showed distant spread. Following external beam therapy 8 of 156 patients had pelvic recurrence. Of these, 2 of 24 were poorly differentiated and 6 of 132 well differentiated. These results reveal no statistically significant difference in terms of local recurrence but metastatic spread is significantly more likely to occur in the poorly differentiated cases.

As previously reported by Joslin et al. [28] the overall 5-year survival for surgery alone, although a few patients had postoperative vaginal therapy, was 67%. This was improved by adding radiotherapy to all stage I cases, with a greater percentage improvement when external beam therapy was added (Fig. 14.1).

Conclusions

For stage I grade I endometrial cancer with evidence of myometrial invasion, surgery with postoperative external beam radiotherapy seems justified. When the myometrium is not invaded, postoperative intravaginal therapy appears to be sufficient.

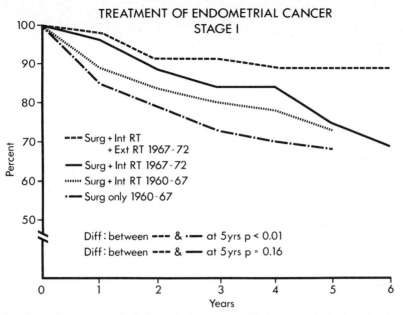

Fig. 14.1. The above graphs indicate the improvement in 5-year survival rates as treatment progresses, from surgery alone (1960–1967) to surgery with postoperative intravaginal irradiation (*Int RT*), and finally surgery with intravaginal and external beam therapy (*Ext RT*).

For stage I grade II and III lesions, preoperative external beam therapy combined with intracavitary treatment appears to produce the best results. This improvement is also reported for stage II cases. However, postoperative external beam radiotherapy with intravaginal treatment also produces comparable results and saves unnecessary surgical delay.

While either preoperative intracavitary or postoperative intravaginal treatment reduces vaginal vault recurrence it does not affect life expectancy. Further progress in firmly establishing the place for external radiotherapy is only likely to be determined as a result of additional controlled clinical trials with separation of the poorly and well differentiated tumours as separate sub-sets.

References

1. Javert CT(1958) Prognosis of endometrial cancer. Obstet Gynecol 30:147–169
2. Regaud C (1922) Influence de la durée d'irradiation sur les effets déterminés dans le testicule par le radium. CR Soc Biol (Paris) 86:787–790
3. Heyman J (1947) Improvement of results in the treatment of uterine cancer JAMA 135:412–416
4. Kottmeier HL (1959) Carcinoma of the corpus uteri; diagnosis and therapy. Am J Obstet Gynecol 78:1127–1140
5. Jones HW (1975) Treatment of adenocarcinoma of the endometrium. Obstet Gynecol Surv 30: 147–169
6. Strickland P (1965) Carcinoma corporis uteri: A radical intracavitary treatment. Clin Radiol 16: 112–118

7. Simon N, Silverstone SM (1976) Afterloading with miniaturized [137] Cs sources in the treatment of cancer of the uterus. Int J Radiat Oncol Biol Phys 1:1017–1021
8. Randall JH, Goddard WB (1956) A study of 531 cases of endometrial carcinoma. Surg Gynecol Obstet 103:221–226
9. Lampe I (1963) Endometrial carcinoma Am J Roentgenol 90:1011–1015
10. Delclos L, Fletcher GH (1969) Malignant tumours of the endometrium: Evaluation of some aspects of radiotherapy. M.D. Anderson Hospital. In: Cancer of the uterus and ovary 11th Clinical conference on cancer. M.D. Anderson Hospital and Tumor Institute, Houston, 1966. Year Book Medical Publishers, Chicago, pp 62–72
11. Lewis BV, Stallworthy JA, Cowdell R (1970) Adenocarcinoma of the body of the uterus. J. Obstet Gynaecol Br Commonw 77:343–348
12. Javert CT (1952) The spread of a benign and malignant endometrium in the lymphatic system with a note on co-existing vascular involvement. Am J Obstet Gynecol 64:780–806
13. Lees DH (1969) An evaluation of treatment in carcinoma of the body of the uterus. J Obstet Gynaecol Br Commonw 76:615–623
14. Shah CA, Green TH (1972) Evaluation of current management of endometrial carcinoma. Obstet Gynecol 39:500–509
15. Lewis BV (1971) Nodal spread in relation to penetration and differentiation. Proc R Soc Med 64:406–407
16. Di Saia PJ, Creasman WT (1981) Clinical gynecologic oncology. CV Mosby, St. Louis, p 144
17. Salazar OM, Feldstein ML, DePapp EW, Bonfiglio TA, Keller BE, Rubin P, Rudolph JM (1978) Management of clinical stage I endometrial carcinoma. Cancer 41:1016–1026
18. Graham J (1971) The value of pre-operative or post-operative treatment by radium for carcinoma of the uterine body. Surg Gynecol Obstet 132:855–860
19. Piver MS (1980) Stage I endometrial carcinoma: The role of adjunctive radiation therapy. Int J Radiat Oncol Biol Phys 6:367–368
20. Kuipers TJ (1981) Personal communication to the European Curietherapy Group
21. Boronow RC (1969) Carcinoma of the corpus: Treatment at M.D. Anderson Hospital, In: Cancer of the uterus and ovary. 11th clinical conference on cancer. M.D. Anderson Hospital and Tumor Institute, Houston, 1966. Year Book Medical Publishers, Chicago, pp 62–72
22. Dally VM (1978) The optimization of radiotherapy in endometrial cancer. In: Brush MG, King RJB, Taylor RW (eds) Endometrial cancer. Ballière Tindall, London, pp 163–178
23. Dobbie BMW (1953) Vaginal recurrences in carcinoma of the body of the uterus and their prevention by radiotherapy. J Obstet Gynaecol Br Commonw 60:702–705
24. Ritcher N, Lucas WE, Yon JL, Sanford GD (1981) Preoperative whole pelvic external irradiation — stage I endometrial cancer. Cancer 48:58–62
25. Gagnon JD, Moss WT, Gabourel LS, Stevens KR (1979) External irradiation in the management of stage II endometrial carcinoma. Cancer 44:1247–1251
26. Onsrud M, Kolstad P, Normann T (1976) Postoperative external pelvic irradiation in carcinoma of the corpus stage I: A controlled clinical trial. Gynecol Oncol 4:222–231
27. Creasman WT, Boronow RC, Morrow CP, Disai PJ, Blessing J (1976) Adenocarcinoma of the endometrium: Its metastatic lymph node potential. Gynecol Oncol 4:239
28. Joslin CA, Vaishampayan GV, Mallik A (1977) The treatment of early cancer of the corpus uteri. Br J Radiol 50:38–45
29. Purcell JL, Underwood PB (1971) Adenocarcinoma of the endometrium: A ten-year experience at the Medical University of South Carolina. South Med J 64:961–966
30. Dobbie BMW, Taylor CW, Waterhouse JAH (1965) A study of carcinoma of the endometrium. J Obstet Gynaecol Br Commonw 72:659–673
31. Rutledge FN, Tan SK, Fletcher GH (1958) Vaginal metastasis from adenocarcinoma of the corpus uteri. Am J Obstet Gynecol 75:164–174
32. Beiler DD, Schmutz DA, O'Rourke TL (1972) Carcinoma of the endometrium: Radiation and surgery versus surgery alone. Radiology 102:159–164
33. Liu W. Meigs JV (1955) Radical hysterectomy and pelvic lymphadenectomy: A review of 473 cases including 244 for primary invasive carcinoma of the cervix. Am J Obstet Gynecol 69:1–32

15 · Recurrence in Endometrial Carcinoma as a Function of Extended Surgical Staging Data

(A Gynaecological Oncology Group Study)

C.P. Morrow, W.T. Creasman, H. Homesley, E. Yordan, R. Park and B. Bundy

Introduction

The Gynecologic Oncology Group (GOG) is a national cooperative study group funded by the National Cancer Institute. On 20 June 1977 the GOG activated Protocol 33 entitled *A Clinical–Pathologic Study of Stage I and II Carcinoma of the Endometrium*. Approximately 30 participating institutions entered 1180 cases in a little less than 6 years. The study was closed to stage I, G1 cases on 8 October 1979 and to all entries on 5 February 1983. Thus it is a non-consecutive series weighted in favour of the G2, G3 lesions.

Materials and Methods

The requirements for entry into the protocol specified that the patients must be clinical (FIGO) stage I or stage II cases with adenocarcinoma and no clinical evidence of cervical involvement. The patients could have no other primary malignancy except for non-melanomatous skin cancer; nor were the entries to have any preoperative radiation therapy, not even remote treatment. Routine preoperative assessment required a chest X-ray and basic laboratory studies. The operative procedure to be carried out on every patient was subtotal pelvic and distal aortic lymph node dissection, pelvic peritoneal cytology, extrafascial abdominal hysterectomy, and bilateral salpingo-oöphorectomy.

Representative histopathology slides of the primary lesion and nodal or adnexal metastases were forwarded from the participating institutions to GOG headquarters for review. The surgico-pathological data collected for each patient included: (a) histological grade (1, 2 or 3) and type; (b) maximum depth of invasion into the myometrium in thirds; (c) extension to the isthmus or cervix; (d) adnexal metastases; (e) pelvic node involvement; (f) high common or aortic node involvement; and (g) pelvic peritoneal cytology. This information, along with demographic and follow-up data, was entered into a computer at the GOG Statistical Office in Buffalo, New York for storage and analysis. The computer data sheets were reviewed by gynaecological oncologists for accuracy.

Results

This preliminary report deals with the 528 patients for whom all surgical staging data (pelvic and aortic node dissection, adnexal resection, and pelvic peritoneal cytology) and at least 2 years of follow-up were available. The frequency with which these risk factors were positive in stage Ia, Ib and II (occult) are presented in Table 15.1. The percentage with aortic and pelvic node involvement increases substantially with each increment in stage; there is no obvious difference in the frequency of adnexal metastases or positive cytology when comparing stage Ib with stage II. When the four risk factors are evaluated relative to histological grade, there is a marked increase in the frequency of 'positiveness' from grade 1 to grade 2 (Table 15.2). This is also true for the degree of myometrial invasion (Table 15.3), which appears to be a more sensitive predictor of risk for extra-uterine spread.

The next four tables (Tables 15.4–15.7) correlate the risk for positive pelvic nodes, aortic nodes, adnexal metastases and positive peritoneal cytology for depth of myometrial penetration within each grade. In general it can be said that the frequency of metastases increases with worsening grade and invasion. For G1 lesions confined to the endometrium, only 1 of 77 cases had pelvic nodal involvement; that single patient had cervical extension. For stage I, grade 1 cases there were 0 of 74 patients without invasion and only 1 of 77 with superficial invasion who had pelvic node metastases. None of these 151 stage I, grade 1 cases had aortic node invasion. On the other hand, when the isthmus or cervix was involved,

Table 15.1. GOG[a] protocol 33: Frequency of positive risk factors versus FIGO stage

FIGO stage		Pelvic nodes (%)	Aortic nodes (%)	Adnexal metastasis (%)	Pelvic cytology (%)
IA	($n = 251$)	8	3	3.5	8
IB	($n = 204$)	12	7	7	14
II (occ[b])	($n = 73$)	20	14	5.5	12
Total	($n = 528$)	11	6	5	10.5

[a] Gynecologic Oncology Group
[b] occ = clinically occult

Table 15.2. GOG protocol 33: Frequency of positive risk factors versus histological grade

Histological grade	Pelvic nodes n (%)	Aortic nodes n (%)	Adnexal metastasis n (%)	Pelvic cytology n (%)
1 (n = 197)	7 (4)	4 (2)	5 (2.5)	11 (5.5)
2 (n = 214)	24 (11)	14 (6)	7 (3.5)	25 (12)
3 (n = 117)	28 (24)	14 (12)	15 (13)	20 (17)
Total (n = 528)	59 (11)	32 (6)	27 (5)	56 (10.5)

Table 15.3. GOG protocol 33: Risk factors versus muscle invasion

Muscle invasion	Pelvic nodes n (%)	Aortic nodes n (%)	Adnexal metastasis n (%)	Pelvic cytology n (%)
None (n = 107)	2 (2)	1 (1)	4 (4)	6 (6)
Inner 1/3 (n = 211)	11 (5)	3 (1.4)	3 (1.5)	19 (8)
Mid 1/3 (n = 89)	11 (12)	6 (7)	8 (9)	11 (12)
Outer 1/3 (n = 121)	35 (29)	22 (18)	12 (10)	21 (17)
Total (n = 528)	59 (11)	32 (6)	27 (5)	57 (11)

Table 15.4. GOG protocol 33: Frequency of pelvic node metastasis versus grade and myometrial invasion

	Muscle invasion			
Histological grade	None n (%)	Inner 1/3 n (%)	Mid 1/3 n (%)	Outer 1/3 n (%)
1	1/77 (1)	2/85 (2)	1/20 (5)	3/15 (20)
2	1/19 (5)	5/91 (5)	7/15 (14)	11/53 (21)
3	0/11 –	4/35 (11)	3/18 (7)	21/53 (40)

Table 15.5. GOG protocol 33: Frequency of aortic node metastasis versus grade and myometrial invasion

	Muscle invasion			
Histological grade	None n (%)	Inner 1/3 n (%)	Mid 1/3 n (%)	Outer 1/3 n (%)
1	0/77 –	0/85 –	2/20 (10)	2/15 (13)
2	1/19 (5)	3/91 (3)	2/51 (4)	8/53 (15)
3	0/11 –	0/38 –	2/18 (11)	12/53 (23)

Table 15.6. GOG protocol 33: Frequency of adnexal metastasis versus grade and myometrial invasion

	Myometrial invasion			
Histological grade	None n (%)	Inner 1/3 n (%)	Mid 1/3 n (%)	Outer 1/3 n (%)
1	1/77 (1)	0/85 –	2/20 (10)	2/15 (13)
2	2/19 (10)	0/91 –	4/51 (8)	1/53 (2)
3	1/11 (9)	3/34 (9)	1/18 (11)	9/53 (17)

i.e. occult stage II, G1, there were 2 of 11 (18.2%) patients with no myometrial invasion or superficial myometrial invasion who had pelvic node metastases. None of the 11 had aortic node spread. At the other end of the spectrum, the grade 3 deeply invasive (outer 1/3) cancers have a 40% rate of pelvic node metastases, 36% in stage I (16/44) and 55% in occult stage II (5/9) while the rate of aortic node metastases for these groups is 18% (8/44) and 44% (4/9) respectively. In all, 22/59 or 37.3% of the cases with pelvic node metastases also had aortic node metastases, an association which increased with worsening disease. The highest rates of nodal metastases within each grade were found in the most deeply invading tumours. Even for stage I, G1 lesions, 20% (2/9) with outer third invasion had pelvic node metastases. For G2 and G3 stage I lesions, there was a 6.2% (5/81) and a 13.3% (4/30) risk of pelvic node metastases with the superficially invasive lesions, while the aortic node risk was largely confined to the more deeply invasive cancers.

The pattern for adnexal metastases (Table 15.6) is less clear, although the highest rate of involvement is in the grade 3, outer 1/3 compartment—17% (9/53). Perhaps of greater significance is the complete absence of adnexal metastases among the 74 grade 1 cases with no myometrial invasion and the 77 grade 1 cases with superficial myometrial invasion, since it is in these categories that most of the cases diagnosed from postoperative vaginal hysterectomy specimens are to be found.

While the highest rate of positive cytology (Table 15.7) was in the group with grade 3, outer 1/3 muscle invasion (22.6%; 12/15), the correlation with invasion of the myometrium and histological grade is even less consistent than that found with adnexal metastases. A surprisingly high percentage of positive pelvic washings occurred among patients with no muscle invasion or only superficial invasion.

In Table 15.8 the two year follow up is summarised. For the entire study group the recurrence rate is 9.7%. Focusing on the effect of the various sites of extra-uterine extension, the recurrence rate for pelvic node involvement only is 4%; aortic node involvement only, 30%; adnexal metastases only, 18%. The recurrence rate for positive pelvic cytology only at 2 years is 14%. If more than one of these sites was involved there was a 43% relapse rate at 2 years while the failure rate for patients with all sites negative was a low 5.5%.

The complications are given in Table 15.9. Although 20% had significant surgical adverse effects, for most of these the risk was probably not altered by the extended surgical procedure. Very important, of course, is the death of one patient for every 200 entries. A substantial number of complications were life threatening and several patients required re-operation.

Table 15.7. GOG protocol 33: Frequency of positive pelvic cytology versus grade and myometrial invasion

| Histological grade | Myometrial invasion | | | |
	None n (%)	Inner 1/3 n (%)	Mid 1/3 n (%)	Outer 1/3 n (%)
1	3/77 (4)	6/85 (6)	1/20 (5)	2/15 (14)
2	1/19 (5)	6/91 (8)	10/51 (20)	7/53 (13)
3	2/11 (8)	6/35 (17)	0/18 –	12/53 (23)

Table 15.8. GOG protocol 33: Tumour recurrence versus risk factors

	n	Recurrence at 2 years (%)
One factor only $\oplus$ [a]		
$\oplus$ Pelvic nodes	26	4
$\oplus$ Aortic nodes	10	30
$\oplus$ Adnexa	11	18
$\oplus$ Pelvic cytology	35	14
Two or more $\oplus$	42	43
All factors $\ominus$ [b]	412	5.5
All cases	536	9.7

[a] $\oplus$ = Positive for metastasis
[b] $\ominus$ = Negative for metastasis

Table 15.9. GOG protocol 33: Complications

	(%)
None	80
Death	0.5
Infection	3.3
Blood loss > 1000 cc	2.5
Gastrointestinal	2.1
Pulmonary embolus	1.2
Lymphocyst	1.2
Evisceration	0.4

Discussion

In 1970 Lewis, Stallworthy and Cowdell [1] reported from England that 11% of 107 women with surgically treated stage I endometrial carcinoma had pelvic lymph node metastases. They also observed that 5/12 patients with nodal metastases survived 5 or more years. In the United States it was widely believed at that time that endometrial cancer, when it invaded the lymphatic system, would metastasise primarily to the aortic lymph nodes, especially those nodes at the level of the renal pedicles. Furthermore, it was believed that involvement of the aortic nodes was invariably fatal, a situation which discouraged any inclination to identify and treat aortic nodal disease. A corollary to this perception of the pathophysiology of endometrial cancer was that pelvic node metastases were a manifestation of advanced corpus cancer. Consequently, it was commonly held that treating the pelvic nodes was also fruitless: if they were not involved by cancer the nodes required no treatment—if metastases were present the treatment would not help.

Despite the significance of the Oxford data relative to the treatment of endometrial carcinoma in vogue in the United States at that time, the report was largely ignored until a collaborative study involving the Universities of Southern California (USC), Mississippi and Duke confirmed the Oxford data [2]. The concordance of the United States and Oxford pelvic lymph node data is remarkable (Tables 15.10, 15.11, 15.12). The figures are similar not just for the overall

Table 15.10. Stage I endometrial carcinoma: Reported frequency of positive risk factors

	n	Pelvic nodes (%)	Aortic nodes (%)
Lewis et al.	102	11.2	N/A[a]
Boronow et al.	222	10.4	7.6
GOG Protocol 33	455	9.7	4.8

[a] Data not available

Table 15.11. Stage I endometrial carcinoma: Frequency of pelvic node metastasis versus histological grade

	n	G1 (%)	G2 (%)	G3 (%)	Total (%)
Lewis et al.	107	5.5	10.0	26.3	11.2
Boronow et al.	222	2.2	11.4	26.8	10.4
GOG protocol 33	455	1.7	10.7	22.2	9.7

Table 15.12. Stage I endometrial carcinoma: Frequency of pelvic node metastasis versus muscle invasion

	n	None (%)	Inner 1/3 (%)	Mid 1/3 (%)	Outer 1/3 (%)	Total (%)
Lewis et al.	107	0.0	0.0	14.3	36.2	11.2
Boronow et al.	222	2.1	5.0	17.6	42.4	10.4
GOG protocol 33	455	0.9	5.3	9.2	28.8	9.7

incidence, but also for the relationship which was found between muscle invasion, histological grade and rate of pelvic node metastases. The USC–Mississippi–Duke study contributed two additional important sets of data. First, most of the 222 patients had a limited aortic node dissection providing direct surgico-pathological information about the incidence of aortic node involvement. Second, it repeated the pelvic cytology study first reported from the Norwegian Radium Hospital by Dahle in 1956 [3]. The frequency of positive pelvic cytology suggested that this could be an important cause of treatment failure and might partly answer the perennial question about the source of vaginal cuff recurrences in endometrial carcinoma.

The findings of this three-institution study were considered to be sufficiently important to justify a group-wide protocol by the GOG to confirm and expand the data. By this time the fear of surgery without preparatory radiation, previously so common among the gynaecologists and radiation therapists in the GOG, had been allayed or dispelled to the point that it was agreed to include patients with a positive endocervical curettage (stage II occult). This present report is quite preliminary since the data are taken from half of the entries and only partially analysed (no data on postoperative treatment or site of failure).

There are several objectives of this current large study. (1) We would like to know if the risk for extra-uterine and extra-pelvic spread can be accurately predicted on the basis of the surgico-pathological data obtained from conventional surgery, i.e. total abdominal hysterectomy, bilateral adnexectomy plus pelvic peritoneal cytology. (2) We wish to know whether extended surgical staging is useful, and, if so, what are the indications based upon the information available intra-operatively. (3) Can survival be improved by extending treatment beyond the pelvis? (4) Can we accurately identify patients who need less treatment, i.e. who do not need pelvic field radiation therapy? (5) If extended surgical staging is useful in defining the best treatment, is it safe?

All these questions cannot be answered on the basis of this preliminary analysis, and perhaps not even after detailed study of the entire 1000 cases. Nevertheless, some observations can be made which are applicable to current practice of endometrial cancer management. Peritoneal cytology is an important risk factor and this simple procedure should be done as a routine in every case. However, there is little information about its incidence or significance following radiation therapy; we do not know how serious positive washings are in G1 cases and we do not know the best way to treat patients with positive cytology, although intra-peritoneal radioactive phosphorus may be effective. The frequency of metastases is sufficiently high to warrant treatment of the pelvic nodes for all G2 and G3 stage I cases with any degree of muscle invasion, and G1 cases with deep muscle invasion. All stage II cases probably need treatment of the pelvic nodes, but our numbers are small (0–5 cases in most subgroups). The most radical change in practice will relate to the aortic nodes. The frequency of involvement of aortic nodes in stage I, G2 with deep (outer 1/3) muscle invasion is 16% (6/37); for G3 cases with mid 1/3 invasion it is 14% (2/14), and for G3 cases with outer 1/3 invasion it is 18% (8/44). These are, of course, rates which would justify routine treatment if the morbidity of extended field radiation were negligible, especially in view of the 70% 2-year recurrence-free survival among the cases in this series with aortic node metastases. However, even restricting aortic node radiation to 40 or 45 Gy (4000 or 4500 rad) can be attended by substantial morbidity. It seems probable then, that a limited aortic node dissection will become a requirement for adequate assessment of the extent of endometrial cancer in patients with deep myometrial invasion documented at surgery.

References

1. Lewis BV, Stallworthy JA, Cowdell R (1970) Adenocarcinoma of the body of the uterus. J. Obstet. Gynaecol. Br. Commonw. 77:343–348
2. Boronow RC, Morrow CP, Creasman WT, DiSaia PJ, Silverberg SG, Miller A, Blessing JA (1984) Surgical staging of endometrial cancer: 1. Clinical-pathologic findings of a prospective study. Obstet. Gynecol. 63:825–838
3. Dahle T (1956) Transtubal spread of tumor cells in carcinoma of the body of the uterus. Surg. Gynecol. Obstet. 103:332–336

Ovary

16 · The Aetiology of Ovarian Cancer

M.S. Baylis, W.J. Henderson, C.G. Pierrepoint and K. Griffiths

Introduction

The estimated number of new notifications of ovarian cancer in 1983 in the United States will be 18 200 with 11 500 women dying from the disease in the same period [1]. New registrations of ovarian cancer in England and Wales in 1974 numbered 4178 and 5 years later, 3784 women had died of the disease. Such data illustrate the poor prognosis associated with this condition, with less than 25% of women expecting to survive 5 years (Fig.16.1). The risk of developing ovarian cancer is similar to that for carcinoma of the cervix, 1 in 80, yet as many women die from ovarian cancer as from the other female genital tract malignancies combined. A factor which gives rise for concern is the increasing incidence of the disease. From 1931 to 1970 in England and Wales the mortality rates per million women rose by 15% each decennium [2]. During the period 1971–1980, however, the rate of increase had plateaued to 6.5% (Fig.16.2).

The diversity of the structure and functions of the ovary results in a great variety of tumours of complex histological origin [3,4].

Tumours of epithelial origin constitute 58% of all ovarian neoplasms and 80–90% of all ovarian carcinomas [5,6]. There is an age specificity for the various histological sub-groups of ovarian malignancy. Sex cord tumours are very rare before the third decade but increase in frequency to the fifth, when their incidence remains constant. Germ cell tumours occur in the 10–50 year old age group, while epithelial tumours rarely appear before the age of 10. They then increase exponentially until 40 years of age and have their highest incidence in women in their early sixties. Varying nomenclature and different histological classifications have made comparative histopathological and epidemiological studies virtually impossible. The fact that more than 70 different types of neoplasms have been described

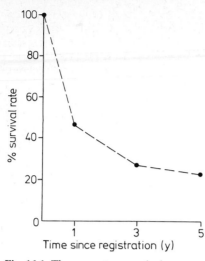

Fig. 16.1. The percentage survival rate over a 5-year period of women registering with ovarian cancer in England and Wales.

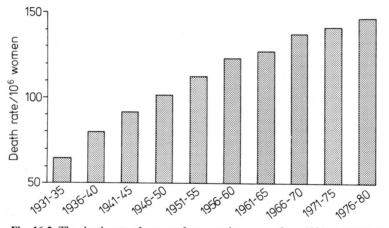

Fig. 16.2. The death rate of women from ovarian cancer from 1931 to 1980 in England and Wales.

highlights the difficulties. The World Health Organisation classification of ovarian tumours [7] should, in future, permit more meaningful comparisons to be undertaken.

Possible Causal Factors

Environmental

Analysis of international mortality rates shows that Northern Europe has four times the incidence rate of Asia [8]. Studies of Japanese migrants living in the

United States [9] show that these Asiatic people exhibit rates of ovarian cancer incidence intermediate between those of their country of origin and their country of adoption. A number of reports have appeared in the literature indicating that certain families show a susceptibility to ovarian malignancy [10] with serous cystadenocarcinomas the most common histological type observed. Prophylactic bilateral oophorectormy has been advocated for these women as soon as they have completed their families, although such an aggressive approach does not guarantee immunity to the development of pelvic cancer, which may exhibit a histological picture similar to that of the ovary and therefore supports the concept of 'generalised instability' of coelomic epithelium. It has been reported that 5%–14% of women with the Peutz-Jeghers syndrome develop ovarian tumours [11,12,13]. Similarly, the basal cell naevus syndrome is associated with the development of ovarian fibromas, although other cell types also occur [14]. The high incidence of ovarian malignancy in the industrialised countries of Northern Europe and North America points strongly to environmental factors playing a significant role in the initiation of the malignant process. A number of studies have shown an association between smoking and the early, spontaneous onset of the menopause [15,16]. There was also a relationship with the level of smoking [17]. Studies of the rodent ovary demonstrated the presence of a non-specific microsomal mono-oxygenase, which metabolises polycyclic aromatic hydrocarbons, present in cigarette smoke and industrial pollutant, to active carcinogenic compounds. Benzo(a)pyrene, also a constituent of cigarette smoke, was found to be toxic to the primordial follicles of rodents and to initial ovarian tumours in mice [18]. Mattison and Thorgeirsson found evidence of a similar microsomal mono-oxygenase system in the human ovary and proposed an association between polycyclic aromatic hydrocarbons and the occurrence of an early menopause in smokers and also a possible carcinogenic role for the induction of ovarian cancer [19]. It is said that the menopause in women occurs when the oocytes are depleted, which normally occurs by the process of atresia [20]. Early ovarian failure may therefore occur if the rate of oocyte loss is accelerated. There is no evidence at present, however, to suggest those women who smoke are more susceptible to ovarian malignancy than non-smokers.

Infectious Diseases

Infectious diseases have been considered as a possible aetiological factor in the causation of ovarian cancer. A higher incidence of rubella infection between the ages of 12 and 18 years in ovarian cancer patients than in controls has been reported [21], whilst there was a lower frequency of mumps [22] and of pneumonia and influenza [23].

Hormonal

It is considered that endogenous hormones play a role in the aetiology of ovarian cancer as, in all international reviews of cancer rates, a strong relationship is known to exist between the incidence of ovarian and breast cancer. Women who develop primary carcinoma of the breast have twice the expected risk of developing a primary ovarian cancer and, vice versa, women with primary ovarian cancer run 3 to 4 times the risk of developing a primary breast malignancy. One hypothesis to explain ovarian epithelial cancer relates growth regulating hormone excess involving the gonadotrophins which act indirectly on the epithelial cells, causing them to replicate following ovulation and cover the denuded surface of the ovary. The epithelium may be incorporated into the stroma of the ovary during the formation of the corpus luteum [24], resulting in inclusion cysts which, because of the multipotentiality of the surface epithelium, may give rise to malignant tumours exhibiting Müllerian cell types [25]. This hypothesis also suggests that the interruption of the normal cyclical control of the ovary by gonadotrophin would be protective and reduce the number of inclusion cysts [26]. This would also account for the rarity of ovarian epithelial neoplasia prior to puberty. A number of case control studies support this concept, showing that pregnancy and lactation have a protective role [23,27,28,29]. Furthermore, in women under 50, incomplete pregnancies were found to be protective, as was the use of oral contraceptives. Beral inversely correlated death from ovarian cancer with the number of children born [30]. It would seem that nulliparous Caucasian women of northern European descent, who live in an industrialised country and who also have a family history of cancer, are at greatest risk of developing epithelial neoplasia of the ovary.

The incidence of breast, endometrial and ovarian cancer was noted by Stadel [31] to be inversely correlated with the dietary intake of iodine, a deficiency which may lead to primary hypothyroidism. Primary hyperthyroidism is associated with elevated prolactin levels [32] and also a 'potentiation' of the effects of gonadotrophins [33], a situation which might lead to excessive oestrogen synthesis and secretion and a possible overall increased risk of ovarian, endometrial and breast malignancy. Biskind and Biskind [34] demonstrated that ovarian tumours of granulosa cell origin could be induced in the rat, probably as a result of excessive gonadotrophin release brought about by castration of the animal and transplantation of part or whole of one ovary into the spleen. As the blood leaving the spleen drains directly to the liver the steroids produced by the transplanted ovary are immediately metabolised and rendered ineffective in the normal feedback of hypothalamus and pituitary. Studies from this Institute [35] confirmed the elevated levels of follicle-stimulating hormone (FSH) and luteinising hormone (LH) following this transplantation procedure. This is an interesting model but is of limited value as granulosa cell tumours are rare in women.

Excessive gonadotrophin stimulation in the rat may also be achieved by immunising with testosterone 3-(O-carboxymethyl imino-bovine serum albumin)-T-3-BSA) [36]. This leads to a grossly elevated, total serum testosterone concentration, with a decrease in free circulating, biologically-active testosterone which is bound by the anti-testosterone antibodies. Exogenous hormones have also been implicated in the aetiology of ovarian cancer [37] in a follow-up survey of 908 women who had received conjugated equine oestrogen postmenopausally. It was also stated that there was a greater risk of developing ovarian cancer in those women who had, in addition, taken stilboestrol.

Talc and Asbestos

It is of interest that those women employed in the rubber, electrical and textile industries are at greater risk of developing ovarian malignancy than those involved in other manufacturing industries [38,39]. The association between asbestos exposure and lung cancer in man was first suggested by Lynch and Smith in 1935 [40]. Further studies confirmed that certain types of asbestos, in addition to their fibrogenic properties, also possessed carcinogenic potential [41]. In 1960, 32 cases of pleural mesothelioma in persons exposed to crocidolite in South Africa were described [42]. Eleven cases of peritoneal tumours associated with asbestos exposure were also reported by Keal [43] and a further nine by Entiknap and Smither [44]. Moreover, Graham and Graham [45] reported the presence of birefringent crystals in human ovarian cancers and related them to asbestos but they were unable to characterise them. Certain ovarian tumours show histological similarity to pleural and peritoneal mesotheliomas. This may be explained by the fact that the ovarian surface epithelium is of mesothelial origin, which confers upon it its unique ability to produce ovarian tumours of multiple cell types including combinations of serous, mucinous, endometrioid, mesonephroid and mesothelial cell types [46].

An extraction replication technique was developed in the Tenovus Institute to investigate foreign particulate material present in biological tissues [47]. This technique was used to investigate and identify various types of contaminating particles in sections of tissue from, for example, the lung and ovaries [48]. It failed to demonstrate the presence of asbestos in human ovaries, as suggested by Graham and Graham, but did establish the presence of talc particles in both normal and neoplastic tissue [49]. Unequivocal identification of individual particles was achieved by using an electron microscope microanalyser (EMMA). There is good evidence that talc may reach the ovary by traversing the female genital tract. Egli and Newton [50] instilled carbon black particles suspended in a 30% dextran solution into the posterior fornix of vaginas of three women undergoing hysterectomy. At laparotomy, in two of the three patients, carbon particules could be found at the fimbrial ostia of the fallopian tube within 40 min of the vaginal instillation. Further confirmation of the migration of particulate material from the vagina to the peritoneal cavity, with uptake into the ovary, was provided by studies using technetium-99 labelled human albumin spheres instilled into the vagina for the purpose of hysterosalpingography by radionuclide scintigraphy [51,52]. Work from this laboratory [53] has shown that when a suspension of talc is introduced either into the posterior aspect of the uterus or even into the vagina of rats, the material can be located in the ovaries within 4 days of the instillation.

Talc is widely used in the pharmaceutical and cosmetic industries and has been used in association with certain types of contraceptive. Many women dust their perinea with talc and some apply it to their sanitary wear [54]. Furthermore, talc particles have been shown to embed in both cultured human lung fibroblasts and in rat ovarian epithelial cells, probably by the process of pinocytosis. Oxygen incineration studies of human ovarian tissue indicated that the amount of talc present could be of the order of 2×10^5 particles per mm^3 [55]. Reports that commercial talcs are contaminated with particles of asbestos [10] have not been substantiated in this Institute, where nearly all forms of natural talc produced from various countries around the world have been analysed. It is well established that talc can induce granulomata in the peritoneal cavity [56] and contamination of the ovary may result in disturbances in the ovarian stroma leading to altered steroid biosynthesis.

In this laboratory, a suspension of asbestos-free Italian 00000 talc in phosphate-buffered saline was injected below the rat ovarian bursa [57]. Within 6 weeks of injection many animals demonstrated cystic changes which, by 1 year, had developed into ovarian bursal cysts, 5 cm or more in diameter (Fig.16.3). Histo-

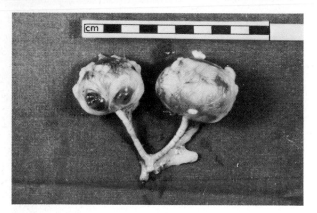

Fig. 16.3. Bilateral ovarian bursal cysts from a rat 12 months after the sub-bursal injection of a suspension of talc.

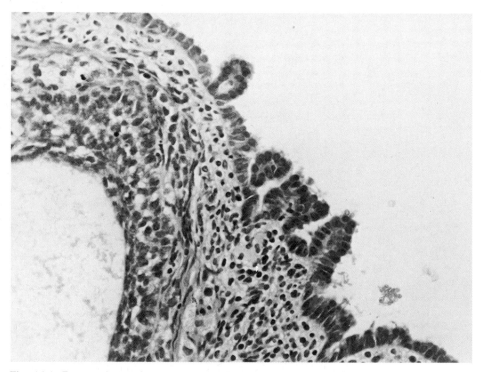

Fig. 16.4. Rat ovarian surface germinal epithelium subsequent to the sub-bursal injection of a suspension of talc. Note papillary formation and the multilayering of the surface epithelium. Stained with H & E. (× 200)

logical examination of these talc-treated ovaries showed multilayering of the surface germinal epithelium (Fig.16.4) with papillary outgrowths, a pathology not inconsistent with preneoplasia and which resembled the histological findings in the ovaries of guinea pigs treated with intraperitoneal asbestos [45]. The possibility that contaminating talc particles may play a role in initiating ovarian dysfunction, which could lead to neoplasia, requires careful consideration. The possible adverse affects of presence of talc in the ovary are being intensively investigated in this Institute. Several different animal species are being used, including the chicken, which is known to have a high incidence of ovarian adenocarcinoma when kept in artificial light [2]. The possibility that talc may act as a co-carcinogen is being examined. Its adsorptive properties are well known and, once located in the ovary, may retain circulating carcinogens for longer periods than normal. Equivalent studies are being carried out in vitro since it has been shown that talc will penetrate epithelial cells in culture and, although transformation of the cells has not been shown, the addition of a chemical such as dimethylbenzanthracene, which does not usually induce ovarian cancer, may well induce such changes.

It certainly cannot be said at present that talc causes ovarian cancer. Its presence in such tumours was unexpected and unwarranted. It is because the cause of ovarian carcinoma is unknown and that talc has a chemical similarity with asbestos that these investigations were instigated.

References

1. Silverberg E (1983) Cancer statistics 1983. CA — A Cancer J Clinicians 33:9
2. Campbell H (1975) In: Brush MG, Taylor RW (eds) Gynaecological malignancy: Clinical and experimental studies. Williams & Wilkins, Baltimore, pp 111–132
3. Wynder EL, Dodo H, Barber HK, (1969) Epidemiology of cancer of the ovary. Cancer 23:352–370
4. Russell P (1979) The pathological assessment of ovarian neoplasms 1. Introduction to the common 'epithelial' tumours and analysis of benign epithelial tumours. Pathology 11:5–26
5. Doll R, Muir C, Waterhouse J (1970) Cancer incidence in five continents. Vol. II Springer, Berlin, pp 29–37
6. Katsube Y, Berg JW, Silverberg SG (1982) Epidemiologic pathology of ovarian tumours: a histopathologic review of primary ovarian neoplasms diagnosed in the Denver Standard Metropolitan Statistical Area, 1 July–31 December 1969 and 1 July–31 December 1979 Int J Gyncecol Pathol 1:3–16
7. Serov SF, Scully RE, Sobin LH (1973) Histological typing of ovarian tumours, No 9 World Health Organisation, Geneva
8. Waterhouse J, Muir C, Correa P, Powell J (1976) Cancer incidence in five continents, Vol III, IARC Scientific Publication No 15. Lyon, pp 453–485
9. Haenszel W, Kurihara M (1968) Studies of Japanese migrants 1. Mortality from cancer and other diseases among Japanese in the United States. J Natl Cancer Inst 40:43–68
10. Lingeman C (1974) Etiology of cancer of the human ovary: A review. J Natl Cancer Inst 53:1603–1618
11. Dozois RR, Kemper RD, Dahlin DC (1970) Ovarian tumours associated with the Peutz-Jeghers syndrome. Ann Surg 172:233–238
12. Scully RE (1970) Sex cord tumour with annular tubules. A distinctive ovarian tumour of the Peutz-Jeghers syndrome. Cancer 25:1107–1121
13. Christian CD (1971) Ovarian tumours: An extension of the Peutz-Jeghers syndrome. Am J Obstet Gynecol 111:529–534

14. Berlin NI (1966) Basal cell naevus syndrome. In: Combined clinicial staff conference at the National Institute of Health. Ann Intern Med 64:403–421
15. Daniel HW (1976) Osteoporosis of the slender smoker. Arch Intern Med 136:298–304
16. Baily A, Robinson D, Vessey M (1977) Smoking and the age of natural menopause. Lancet II:722
17. Jick H, Porter J, Norrison AS (1977) Relation between smoking and age of natural menopause. Lancet I:1354–1355
18. Jull JW (1973) In: Busch J (ed) Methods in Cancer Research. Academic, New York, Vol VII, pp 131–186
19. Mattison DR, Thorgeirsson L (1978) Smoking and industrial pollution and their effects on the menopause and ovarian cancer. Lancet I:187–188
20. Ingram DL (1962) In: Zuckerman S (ed) The ovary. Academic, New York, Vol I, pp 247–273
21. McGowan L, Parent L, Lednar W, Norris HJ (1979) The women at risk of developing ovarian cancer. Gynecol Oncol 7:325–344
22. West RO (1966) Epidemiologic study of malignancies of the ovaries. Cancer 19:1001–1007
23. Joly DJ, Lillienfeld AM, Diamond EL, Brass IDJ (1974) An epidemiologic study of the relationship of reproductive experience to cancer of the ovary. Am J Epidemiol 99:190–209
24. Radisavljevic SA (1977) The pathogenesis of ovarian inclusion cysts and cystomas. Obstet Gynecol 49:424–429
25. Hertig AT, Gore H (1961) Tumours of the female sex organs, Part 3 Armed Forces Institute of Pathology, Washington, DC, p 76
26. Fathalla MF (1971) Incessant ovulation — A factor in ovarian neoplasia. Lancet I:163
27. Newhouse ML, Pearson RM, Fullerton JM, Boresfen FAM, Shannon MS (1977) A case control study of carcinoma of the ovary. Br J Prev Soc Med 31:148–153
28. Annegers JF, Strom H, Decker DG, Dockerty MD, O'Fallon WM (1979) Ovarian Cancer: Incidence and case-control study. Cancer 43:723–729
29. Casagrande JT, Louie EW, Pike MC, Roy S, Ross RK, Henderson Be, (1979) 'Incessant ovulation' and ovarian cancer. Lancet II:170–172
30. Beral V, Fraser P, Chivers C (1978) Does pregnancy protect against ovarian cancer? Lancet I:1083–1086
31. Stadel BV (1976) Dietary iodine and the risk of breast, endometrial and ovarian cancer. Lancet I:890–891
32. Ingbar SJ, Woebar KA (1974) In: Williams RH (ed) Textbook of endocrinology 5th ed. Saunders, Philadelphia, pp 95–232
33. Longcope C (1975) Breast cancer and estriol dynamics: Program of the Breast Cancer Task Force. National Cancer Institute, National Institute of Health, Washington.
34. Biskind MS, Biskind GR (1944) Development of tumours in the rat ovary after transplantation into the spleen. Proc Soc Exp Biol Med 55:176–179
35. Seager SE, Boyns AR, Blumgart LM (1974) Histological and hormonal studies in rats bearing ovarian implants in the spleen. Effects of portocaval anastamosis. Eur J Cancer 10:35–40
36. Hillier SG, Groom GV, Boyns AR, Cameron EHD (1974) Development of polycystic ovaries in rats actively immunised against T-3-BSA. Nature 250:433–434
37. Hoover R, Fraumeni JF, Gray LA (1977) Stilbeostrol (Diethylstiboestrol) and the risk of ovarian cancer. Lancet II:533–534
38. Manusco TF (1975) In: Levinson C (ed) The new multinational health hazards. International Chemical Foundation, Geneva 80
39. Campbell JG (1969) Tumours of the fowl. Heinemann Medical, London pp 171–200
40. Lynch KM, Smith WA (1935) Carcinoma of the lung in asbestos silicosis. Am J Cancer 24:56–61
41. Doll R (1955) Mortality from lung cancer in asbestos workers. Br J Ind Med 12:81–86
42. Wagner JC, Sleggs CA, Marchand P (1960) Diffuse pleural mesothelioma and asbestos exposure in North-Western Cape Province. Br J Ind Med 17:260–271
43. Keal EE (1960) Asbestosis and abdominal neoplasms. Lancet II:1211–1216
44. Entiknap JB, Smither J (1964) Peritoneal tumours in asbestosis. Br J Ind Med 21:20–31
45. Graham J, Graham R (1967) Ovarian cancer and asbestos. Environ Res 1:115–128
46. Parmley TH, Woodruff JD (1974) The ovarian mesothelioma. Am J Obstet Gynecol 120:234–241
47. Henderson WJ (1969) A simple replication technique for the study of biological tissues by electron microscopy. J Microsc 89:369–372
48. Henderson WJ, Gough J, Harse J (1970) Identification of mineral particles in pneumoconiotic lungs. J Clin Pathol 23:104–109
49. Henderson WJ, Joslin CAF, Turnbull AC, Griffiths K (1971) Talc and carcinoma of the ovary and cervix. J Obstet Gynecol Br Commonw 78:266–272
50. Egli GE, Newton M (1961) The transport of carbon particles in the human female reproductive tract. Fertil Steril 12:151–155

51. Venter PF, Iturralde M (1979) Migration of a particulate radioactive tracer from the vagina to the peritoneal cavity and ovaries. S Afr Med J 55:917–919

52. Iturralde M, Venter PF (1981) Hysterosalpingo-radionuclide scintigraphy (HERS) Semin Nucl Med 11:301–314

53. Baylis MS. Hamilton TC, Henderson WJ, Pierrepoint CG, Griffiths K (to be published) The demonstration of the migration of talc from the vagina and posterior uterus to the ovary in the rat. Environ Res

54. Cramer DW, Welch WR, Scully RE, Wojciechowski CA (1982) Ovarian cancer and talc. Cancer 50:372–376

55. Henderson WJ, Melville-Jones C, Wilson DW, Griffiths K (1978) Oxygen incineration and electron microscope X-ray microanalysis of mineral particles in biological tissues. J Histochem Cytochem 26:1087–1093

56. Lichtman AL, McDonald R, Dixon CF, Mann FC (1946) Talc granuloma. Surg Gynecol Obstet 83:531–558

57. Hamilton TC, Fox H, Buckley H, Henderson WJ, Griffiths K (1984) The effect of talc on the rat ovary. Br J Exp Pathol 65:101–106

17 · Epithelial Ovarian Carcinoma of Low Malignant Potential

D. Barnhill, P. Heller, P. Brzozowski, H. Advani, R. Park,
E. Weiser, W. Hoskins and D. Gallup

Introduction

The American Cancer Society suggested that, in 1983, 18 200 cases of ovarian carcinoma would be discovered in the United States. Early diagnosis is rare, but this disease spreads from the ovaries in a predictable fashion and the majority of these cases will be reported as stage III or stage IV disease. In 1929, Taylor [1] reported a series of ovarian tumours that appeared malignant but behaved in a benign manner. His concept was not immediately accepted. In 1961, the International Federation of Gynecologists and Obstetricians (FIGO) suggested a classification dividing epithelial ovarian tumours into benign, those of proliferative activity, and tumours with clearly malignant characteristics. This classification system became effective in January 1971. The World Health Organization (WHO) followed with a similar categorisation in 1973 [2].

It is now realised that about 15% of epithelial ovarian malignancies are of borderline malignant potential [3]. It has been reported that epithelial ovarian carcinoma of low malignant potential occurs in patients of a younger age than that of patients with frankly invasive ovarian malignancy, and a higher percentage are discovered as stage I. Until recently, treatment modalities for these tumours have paralleled those for invasive carcinoma. This has included surgery with adjuvant radiation and/or chemotherapy. A review by Julian and Woodruff in 1972 suggested that the 5-year survival rate for this group was 83% regardless of stage or adjunctive therapy [4].

This paper retrospectively characterises and reviews the treatment and outcome of a group of patients having known epithelial ovarian tumours of borderline malignant potential.

Materials and Methods

From June 1965 through December 1982, 94 patients with epithelial ovarian tumours of borderline malignant potential were diagnosed and treated at three affiliated institutions of the Uniformed Services University of the Health Sciences, Bethesda, Maryland (Walter Reed Army Center, Naval Hospital, Bethesda, Maryland and Naval Hospital, Portsmouth, Virginia). A review of microscopic sections from each of the 94 tumours confirmed that these lesions had borderline malignant potential, and a retrospective analysis of the treatment and survival of these patients was performed. All tumours were of either serous or mucinous histology.

Microscopic criteria used to define tumours of borderline malignant potential have been outlined by several authors [3,5–11]. Serous tumours were classified as having borderline malignant potential [3,5,6,8] by lack of stromal invasion, including the absence of irregular or destructive invasion with fibrous reaction. Marked complex proliferation of the lining epithelium, including the formation of papillary fronds with or without cribriform pattern, was a characteristic. Stratification of the lining epithelium (the number of cell layers were not identified because its significance is not known), detachment of papillary buds from the lining epithelium and mild to moderate nuclear atypia, were used to distinguish these tumours as being of low malignant potential. The mucinous tumours of borderline malignant potential were identified in a fashion similar to the serous tumours [3,5,6,7,12,13]. The traits used to characterise mucinous tumours are [3,7,12,13] absence of stromal invasion (which is difficult to assess within this histological type), stratification of epithelial tissue between two and three layers [12,13] (four or more layers was considered malignant), mild to moderate nuclear atypia, and papillary infolding of the lining epithelium with budding and bridging.

All patients underwent exploratory laparotomy. Eighty-four patients had total abdominal hysterectomy and bilateral salpingo-oophorectomy. Ten patients had unilateral salpingo-oophorectomy. Adjunctive postoperative therapy, when used, included radiation therapy, chemotherapy, or a combination of radiation therapy and chemotherapy.

Results

The age range of the patients was 18 to 71 years. The median age was 38 years with a mean age of 40 years (SD±13.5). Forty-seven patients (50%) had stage I disease, 13 (14%) had stage II, 33 (35%) had stage III, and 1 (1%) had stage IV

Table 17.1. Distribution of stage and adjuvant therapy in patients with epithelial ovarian tumours of borderline malignant potential

Stage	No adjuvant therapy	Chemotherapy	Radiation therapy	Radiation therapy plus chemotherapy
I	24	13	9	1
II	1	4	5	3
III	–	18	13	2
IV	–	–	–	1

disease. Histologically, 17 of the 94 tumours (18%) were of mucinous type and the remaining 77 (82%) were serous.

Twenty-five patients (27%) received no adjuvant therapy, 27 (29%) received postoperative radiation therapy, 35 (37%) received single or multiagent cytotoxic chemotherapy, and 7 (7%) received postoperative radiation therapy and chemotherapy. The treatment groups were dissimilar, preventing valid statistical analysis. Of patients with stage 1 disease, 24 (51%) received no further therapy, and 23 (49%) received postoperative adjuvant therapy. Of stage II patients, 1 (8%) received no further therapy, and 12 (92%) received adjuvant therapy. All patients with stage III and IV disease received postoperative adjuvant therapy (Table 17.1).

Two patients died from their disease. Both had stage III mucinous tumours. One received radiation therapy and died at 32 months; the other received chemotherapy and survived 9 months. Two patients died from unrelated causes during the study period. Five patients are alive with clinically evident disease (Table 17.2). The remainder of the patients are clinically free of disease at this time. Using the actuarial method of Berkson and Gage, the 5- and 10-year survival rates for the entire study group are 95% and 87%, respectively (Fig. 17.1). The 5-year survival rates for patients treated with postoperative radiation therapy or chemotherapy were 95% and 91%, respectively (Fig. 17.2). Survival appears to favour the patients with serous tumours (Fig. 17.3).

Table 17.2. Patients alive with clinical evidence of disease

Patient	Tumour histology	Stage	Adjuvant therapy	Time from diagnosis (months)
1	Serous	III	Chemotherapy and radiotherapy	136
2	Serous	III	Chemotherapy and radiotherapy	87
3	Serous	III	Chemotherapy	27
4	Serous	III	Chemotherapy	22
5	Serous	III	Chemotherapy	6

Discussion

Aure in 1971 retrospectively reviewed 990 cases of epithelial ovarian carcinoma of which 161 were identified as tumours of borderline malignant potential [14]. The mean age of the patients with true invasive carcinoma was 53 years, but that of patients with tumours of borderline malignant potential was 46. In that study, the 5-year survival for patients with overtly malignant lesions was less than 30% for serous types and 40% for those with mucinous histology. The 10-year survival was poorer in both instances. As in the present study, the serous and mucinous borderline tumours of low malignant potential had a 5-year survival of greater than 90% while the 10-year survival was slightly above (serous) or slightly below (mucinous) 90%. Aure noted that about 80% of the tumours of borderline

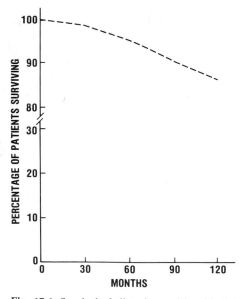

Fig. 17.1. Survival of all patients with epithelial ovarian carcinoma of low malignant potential.

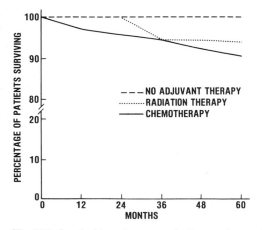

Fig. 17.2. Survival based on type of adjuvant therapy in patients with epithelial ovarian carcinoma of low malignant potential.

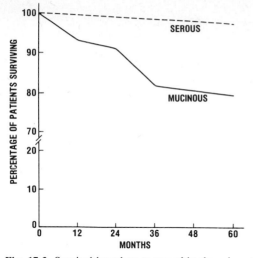

Fig. 17.3. Survival based on tumour histology in patients with epithelial ovarian carcinoma of low malignant potential.

malignant potential were stage I while approximately 30% of the true carcinomas presented at this stage. The present series found only 50% of the patients as stage I. This may be related to more extensive surgical staging performed in recent years. Aure found that 50% of the borderline malignant potential tumours were mucinous while 46% were serous and 4% endometrioid. The present review reports 82% of the cases to be of serous histology while 18% were mucinous.

The following year Julian and Woodruff reviewed 64 cases of low grade papillary serous cystadenocarcinoma [4]. While mean age was not recorded for their series, 68% of the patients were between 21 and 50 years. Their study found that 53% of the cases presented as stage I, while 22% were stage II, and 25% were stage III or IV. This is in agreement with information reported in the present review. In the study by Julian and Woodruff, treatment was not standardised; however, most patients were treated by surgery without postoperative adjunctive therapy. In the present series no adjuvant therapy was received by 25 patients (27%) while 69 patients (73%) received adjuvant treatment. The percentage of patients who received adjuvant therapy in our study increased with advancing stage (Table 17.1). Julian reported a relative 5-year survival of 92% with an absolute survival of 83%. Four patients died of their tumours, 3 were living with tumour, and 4 died of unrelated causes. The present study noted a 95% 5-year survival, while 2 patients died of tumour, 3 patients are alive with evidence of disease and 2 patients died of causes not related to their tumours.

Nikrui in 1981 analysed 62 cases of borderline epithelial tumours of the ovary [15]. The average age of the patients was 54 years with a range of 18 to 90. The present study was at variance with a mean age of 40 years and a median age of 38. Nikrui found that 71% of the tumours occurred as stage I, 10% as stage II, 10% as stage III and IV, and 10% were unstaged or recurrent. The histological distribution of that review revealed 58% to be serous, 40% to be mucinous and 2% to be endometrioid. The present study reveals similar information. A majority of the tumours were stage I. In Nikrui's review 35% of the patients had adjuvant chemotherapy, radiation or a combination following surgical removal of the tumour. The addition of radiation or chemotherapy occurred least in stage I (16%) and most extensively in stage III, IV or recurrent cases (92%). This agrees with the trend of the present study. Nikrui noted that 4 patients died of tumour after recurrence but reported an actuarial 5-year survival of 91% for serous tumours and 81% for mucinous tumours (excepting the recurrent cases). Survival in the present study is equivalent to Nikrui's but does include patients who died of their tumours.

Conclusions

The present series, which has been reported elsewhere [16], and reviews by other authors confirm the fact that epithelial ovarian tumours of borderline malignant potential occur at an earlier age and stage than their invasive counterparts. Survival is similar to that reported by others and is excellent regardless of stage. Surgery alone may be adequate therapy for all stages of this disease. Efficacy of adjuvant therapy is not proven. It is suggested that a prospective randomised study be performed to address the question of adjuvant therapy in treatment of epithelial ovarian tumours of borderline malignant potential.

References

 1. Taylor HC (1929) Malignant and semimalignant tumors of the ovary. Surg Gynecol Obstet 48:204–230
 2. Serov SF, Scully RE, Sobin LH (1973) International histological classification of tumors, No. 9 Histological typing of ovarian tumors. World Health Organization, Geneva, pp 10–21
 3. Colgan TJ, Norris JH (1983) Ovarian epithelial tumors of low malignant potential: A review, Int J Gynecol Pathol 1:367–381
 4. Julian CG, Woodruff JD (1972) The biologic behavior of low-grade papillary serous carcinoma of the ovary. Obstet Gynecol 40:860–867
 5. Katzenstein AA, Mazur MT, Morgan TE, Kao M (1978) Proliferative serous tumors of the ovary. Am J Surg Pathol 2:339–355
 6. Russel P (1979) The pathological assessment of ovarian neoplasms II: Introduction to the common 'epithelial' tumors. Pathology 11:252–282
 7. Scully RE (1979) Tumors of the ovary and maldeveloped gonads. In Atlas of tumor pathology. Armed Forces Institute of Pathology, Washington, DC. fasicle 16, 2nd series, pp 83–91
 8. Novak ER, Woodruff JD (1979) Gynecologic and obstetric pathology. Saunders, Philadelphia, p 406
 9. Russel P (1979) The pathological assessment of ovarian neoplasms I: Introduction to the common 'epithelial' tumors and analysis of benign 'epithelial' tumors. Pathology 11:5–26
10. Russel P, Perkur H (1979) Proliferating ovarian 'epithelial' tumors: a clinicopathological analysis of 144 cases. Aust NZ J Obstet Gynaecol 19:45–51
11. Dallenbach F, Komitowski D (1982) Digital picture analysis of borderline papillary serous cystadenomas of the ovary. In: Dallenbach-Hellweg G (ed) Ovarialtumoren, Vienna. Springer, New York, pp 158–166

12. Hart WR (1977) Ovarian epithelial tumors of borderline malignancy (carcinomas of low malignant potential), Hum Pathol 8:541–549
13. Hart WR, Norris HJ (1973) Borderline and malignant mucinous tumors of the ovary. Cancer 31:1031–1044
14. Aure JC, Hoeg K, Kolstad P (1971) Clinical and histologic studies of ovarian carcinoma. Obstet Gynecol 37:1–9
15. Nikrui N (1981) Survey of clinical behavior of patients with borderline epithelial tumors of the ovary. Gynecol Oncol 12:107–119
15. Nikrui N (1981) Survey of clinical behavior of patients with borderline epithelial tumors of the ovary. Gynecol Oncol 12:107–119
16. Barnhill D, Heller P, Brzozowski P, Advani H, Gallup D (1985) Epithelial ovarian carcinoma of low malignant potential. Obstet Gynecol 65:53–59

18 · The Canadian Ovarian Cancer Trial — Preliminary Results

J.A. Carmichael

Background to the Trials

The Canadian Cancer Society is a voluntary organisation which annually raises approximately 60 million dollars in contributions from the private sector. Approximately 50% of this sum supports the National Cancer Institute of Canada (NCIC), which in turn supports cancer research, mostly in university medical centres throughout the country, as well as an epidemiological division at the University of Toronto and a Clinical Trials Division at Queen's University in Kingston, Ontario. The remaining funds are dedicated to society activities such as education and patient services.

Since 1974 the National Cancer Institute of Canada has conducted a number of prospective randomised clinical trials for carcinoma of the ovary of epithelial origin. This paper will review some of these trials, particularly the current trial (Ov 4) and briefly outline the proposals for the new ovarian trial (Ov 5) to be initiated in the summer of 1984.

Participation in the clinical trials is on a voluntary basis and most university medical centres in the country are contributors (Table 18.1). Clinical protocols are developed by subcommittees of the National Cancer Institute of Canada Clinical Trials Committee. Members of the subcommittee are selected from centres participating, or interested in participating, in that particular clinical trial, and individuals with a particular interest and expertise in these subjects. Attention is also paid to regional and geographical representation.

In Canada great distances are a problem. For those not familiar with the geography of our country, the United Kingdom from Lands End to the Orkneys could be comfortably tucked into the Province of Saskatchewan, and for our American friends, the Lone Star State of Texas could be hidden comfortably in

Table 18.1. NCIC ovarian cancer trial, Ov 4. Contributing centres

Centre	No. of patients
Halifax, N.S.	46
St. John, N.B.	2
Quebec, P.Q.	32
Montreal, P.Q.	6
Kingston, Ont.	31
Ottawa, Ont.	8
Hamilton, Ont.	20
Windsor, Ont.	7
Winnipeg, Man.	54
Saskatoon, Sask.	7
Edmonton, Alta	13
Victoria, B.C.	25
	251

the northern regions of either of the Provinces of Ontario or Quebec. Such vast distances contribute to varying and strongly held differences of clinical opinion, as well as having some considerable bearing on the treatment programmes available for the many patients who travel long distances to the nearest treatment centre.

First Three Trials

The first ovarian trial (Ov 1) was begun in 1974. This was a simple comparison, in patients with advanced ovarian carcinoma, of combination versus sequential chemotherapy, using the most effective drugs available at the time, i.e. melphalan, 5–fluorouracil and methotrexate, in that sequence. Survival rates were identical (Fig. 18.1) and 80% of all patients were dead within 2 years. The results of this trial were published in detail elsewhere [1].

The second ovarian trial (Ov 2) was initiated in 1975. This was a stage 1 'high risk' and stage 2 trial. Following total abdominal hysterectomy, bilateral salpingo-oophorectomy and postoperative pelvic irradiation, patients were randomised to one of three régimes: (1) melphalan for 18 months; (2) intraperitoneal chromic phosphate; or (3) total abdominal irradiation. This trial will have completed accrual by the spring of 1984. The overall survival rate is shown in Fig. 18.2. Early in the trial the chromic phosphate régime was dropped because of a high and serious complication rate. There is to date no difference between the survival rates of the remaining two treatments.

In 1978 the third ovarian trial (Ov 3) for stages 3 and 4 was initiated. At that time melphalan was still considered the most efficient single alkylating agent for epithelial carcinoma of the ovary and the concept of this trial was an attempt to 'consolidate' the tumour with melphalan for six courses and then randomise the patients between melphalan alone and a combination of hexamethylmelamine, adriamycin and melphalan. Shortly after its initiation, this trial had to be aborted. Combinations of the newer agents cisplatinum and adriamycin had demonstrated significantly improved initial response rates and it was the opinion of many members of the Ovary Subcommittee that a national trial should be developed with these agents as first-line chemotherapy.

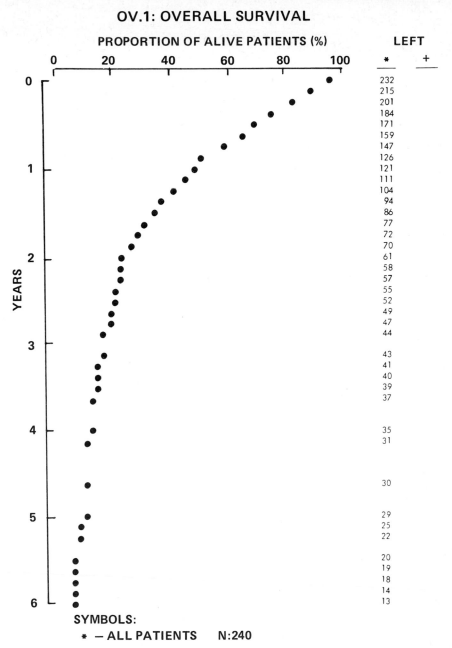

Fig. 18.1. Overall survival of all patients entered into the first Canadian ovarian carcinoma trial, comparing melphalan, 5-fluorouracil and methotrexate in combination, with the same three drugs in sequence.

OVARIAN CARCINOMA TRIAL 2:
STAGES I, II & IIIO – OVERALL SURVIVAL

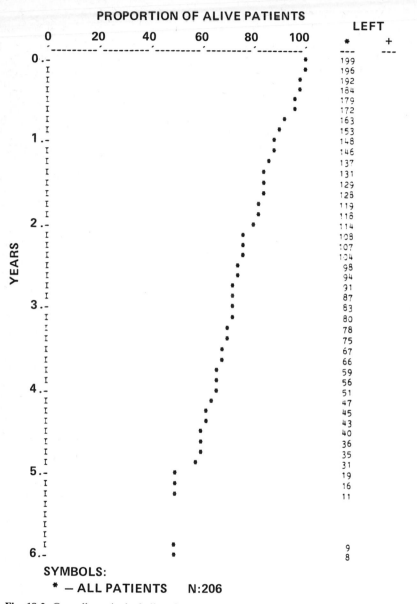

SYMBOLS:

* – ALL PATIENTS   N:206

Fig. 18.2. Overall survival of all patients entered into the second Canadian ovarian carcinoma trial comparing, in patients with 'high risk' stage I and stage II disease, the effects of postoperative treatment with melphalan, intraperitoneal ^{32}P or total abdominal irradiation.

Current Trial

In 1980, therefore, a fourth ovarian trial (Ov 4) was initiated for stages III and IV. Following maximum tumour reductive surgery, all patients are placed on the combination of adriamycin and cisplatinum (50 mg/m² each) at 3- to 4-week intervals for a total adriamycin dose of 450 mg/m². Patients who progress, or who have clinical evidence of disease, or positive second-look surgery at the completion of their adriamycin/cisplatinum programme, are randomised between melphalan and melphalan/hexamethylmelamine. Negative second-look patients are followed only. The overall survival rate at 2 years is 40% (Fig. 18.3). This is double the 2-year survival rate for the first ovary trial (Ov 1).

Table 18.2 outlines the response to adriamycin/cisplatinum in 151 assessable patients. The complete response rate (negative second-look) was 16% (24 patients). This group is being followed only. Of the 24 patients 3 have relapsed, all of whom had residual disease measuring 2–10 cm at the start of chemotherapy.

Table 18.3 shows response by stage and by diameter of residual disease (after surgery). Response related to diameter of residual size suggests three groups: (1) microscopic residual disease; (2) residual disease to 10 cm; and (3) residual disease greater than 10 cm. This very initial impression appears to be holding.

Table 18.2. Response to adriamycin and cisplatinum (total of 151 assessable patients)

Randomised to secondary chemotherapy	109
Had negative 2nd-look	24
Not randomised when disease progressed or after 2nd-look laparotomy	7
Died of progressive disease or toxicity prior to randomisation	11
Overall response	*No. (%)*
Complete response	24 (16)
Partial response	62 (41)
No change	29 (19)
Progressive disease	36 (24)

Table 18.3. Response to adriamycin and cisplatinum by stage and by diameter of residual disease[a]

	Total	CR	PR	NC	PD
Response by stage					
Stage III	123(100)*	22(18)	49(40)	21(17)	31(25)
Stage IV	28(100)	2(7)	13(46)	8(29)	5(18)
Response by diameter of residual disease					
Microscopic	12(100)	6(50)	1(8)	4(33)	1(8)
< 2 cm	41(100)	6(15)	15(37)	7(17)	13(32)
2–10 cm	57(100)	12(21)	24(42)	9(16)	12(21)
> 10 cm	40(100)	0(0)	21(52)	9(23)	10(25)
Unknown	1(100)		1(100)		

[a] Numbers in parentheses represent percentages.
   CR – complete response
   PR – partial response
   NC – no change
   PD – progressive disease

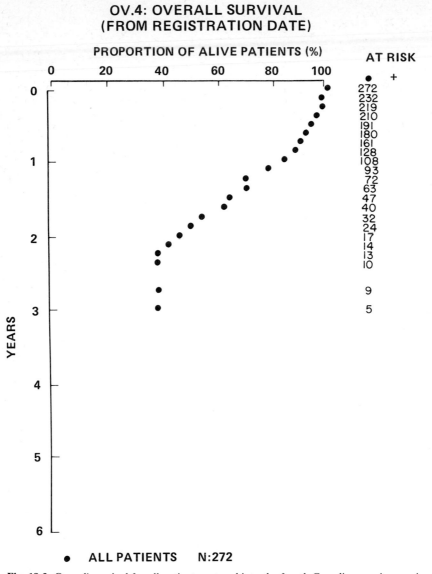

Fig. 18.3. Overall survival for all patients entered into the fourth Canadian ovarian carcinoma trial. Patients who progressed on adriamycin plus cisplatinum were randomised to melphalan or melphalan plus hexamethylmelamine.

OV.4: OVERALL SURVIVAL OF RANDOMIZED
PATIENTS (FROM RANDOMIZATION DATE)

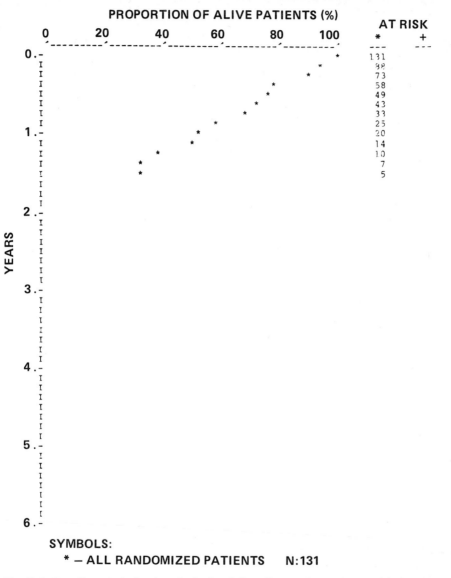

SYMBOLS:
* – ALL RANDOMIZED PATIENTS   N:131

Fig. 18.4. Overall survival of patients in the fourth Canadian ovarian carcinoma trial who progressed on adriamycin plus cisplatinum, and were then randomised to melphalan or melphalan plus hexamethylmelamine.

Further preliminary review of this material suggests that tumour diameter is a more accurate prognosticator of second-look status than either tumour grade or tumour cell type.

Response to second-line chemotherapy, melphalan or melphalan plus hexamethylmelamine, is disappointing (Fig. 18.4). These results are similar to those with melphalan alone as first-line chemotherapy, experienced in the first ovarian trial (Ov 1).

Both current ovary trials (Ov 2 and Ov 4) will complete patient accrual by the spring of 1984. This will allow the Ovarian Subcommittee to consider a new protocol which encompasses all epithelial tumours and all stages in a potential single trial which will recognise not only the importance of clinical staging, but the impact of cell type, degree of differentiation and residual tumour. The new ovary trial (Ov 5) will incorporate all stages and will be structured on precise surgical staging and amount of residual disease. Degree of differentiation and cell type will not be determinants of therapeutic programmes, but will be identified in the analysis of results.

Such a treatment protocol will, we hope, allow a panoramic view of epithelial carcinoma of the ovary, allow a shift of treatment régimes as experience dictates, from more advanced groups to earlier groups, and allow an opportunity for new treatments and even phase 2 studies to be introduced from time to time.

Reference

1. Miller AB, Klassen DJ, Boyes DA et al. (1980) Combinations vs sequential therapy with melphalan, 5-fluorouracil and methotrexate for advanced ovarian cancer. Can Med Assoc J 123:365–371

19 · Second-Look Laparotomy in Stage III Epithelial Ovarian Cancer*

J.S. Berek, N.F. Hacker, L.D. Lagasse, T. Poth, B. Resnick and K. Nieberg

Introduction

The primary management of most patients with ovarian carcinoma involves an initial exploratory laparotomy for staging of early disease and cytoreductive surgery in advanced disease, followed by a planned course of chemotherapy. Since no reliable serum assay or X-ray test is available to monitor the amount of residual disease, an exploratory laparotomy is often performed in patients who are clinically free of disease at the completion of their chemotherapy. This procedure has been termed a second-look operation [1].

The nomenclature of secondary laparotomies for ovarian cancer has not been standardised. The term second-look has been used to describe a secondary laparotomy performed on patients with ovarian cancer for a variety of reasons, including operation for tumour resection in patients with obvious disease progression or bowel obstruction [2]. For our analysis, we use the definition only for those operations performed on patients who are clinically free of disease following a prescribed course of chemotherapy.

Previous reports have concentrated on patient survival based on the findings at second-look [1-8]. Variables associated with each individual patient, such as age, tumour grade, the extent of residual disease at the completion of primary surgery, the type and number of cycles of chemotherapy, the size of the primary and metastatic tumours, the presence of ascites, and the extent of primary cytoreductive surgery have not been thoroughly analysed to determine to what extent they are associated with the findings at second-look laparotomy.

* Reprinted with permission of the American College of Obstetricians and Gynecologists and the publishers of the journal *Obstetrics and Gynecology* (1983) 61:189

Because surgical and chemotherapeutic treatments for epithelial ovarian cancer have been heterogeneous over the past decade, we have chosen to evaluate only our recent 5-year experience for this analysis. The method employed for the second-look operations has been uniform over this period.

Materials and Methods

During a 5-year period, from 1977 to 1982, 228 laparotomies were performed on patients with epithelial ovarian cancers. Of these laparotomies 56 were performed to assess therapeutic response in patients with stage III disease who were clinically free of disease after primary chemotherapy. A negative second-look laparotomy is defined as one which occurs in a patient who has no histological or cytological evidence of tumour at the time of the surgery.

Of the 56 cases, 47 tumours were serous carcinomas, 3 mucinous, 3 endometrioid, and 3 undifferentiated. Using established criteria for grading [9], 12 were grade 1 carcinomas, 24 grade 2, 15 grade 3, and 4 grade 4. Patients with neoplasms of low malignant potential were excluded from this evaluation.

Treatment consisted of chemotherapy in all patients, and all had undergone primary cytoreductive surgery [10] at the UCLA (University of California–Los Angeles) Medical Center (47 cases) or prior to referral (9 cases).

If macroscopic tumour is discovered, it is our policy to attempt secondary cytoreductive surgery, if optimal resection is considered feasible [11]. If no macroscopic disease is visualised, a thorough and systematic sampling of tissues is undertaken. Following the aspiration of any free peritoneal fluid, which is submitted separately for cytological evaluation, multiple intraperitoneal washings using about 50 cc of normal saline are instilled and recovered in five separate locations: the pelvic cul-de-sac, the right and left paracolic gutters, and each hemidiaphragm. Multiple separate biopsies of the peritoneal surfaces are taken at any site of previously documented tumour, the pedicles of the infundibulopelvic ligaments, the pelvic cul-de-sac, the bladder dome peritoneum, the pelvic side walls, both paracolic gutters, and any irregular surface elevations or suspicious areas. At lease 20 biopsies are taken. A Pap smear or biopsy is taken of the right hemidiaphragm. A thorough lymph node sampling of the pelvic and periaortic lymph nodes below the level of the inferior mesenteric vessels is performed. Residual omentum, if present, is removed from the greater curvature of the stomach. The entire length of the bowel and its mesentery is inspected and palpated. If any single biopsy or cytological specimen reveals evidence of malignancy, the procedure is termed 'positive'.

Using Fisher's exact test, some of these categorical variables were significantly different from expectation. The logarithmic transformation of the significant variables were used in a discriminant analysis to determine which of these variables could properly classify the patients into either negative or positive second-look groups. The variables were stepped into the function according to which variables added the most to the separation of the second-look groups, a procedure based on the F statistic, which is adjusted to reduce bias in the classification of the second-look groups [12].

Results

Of 56 patients 18 (32.1%) had a negative second-look laparotomy. All patients without documented tumour received no further treatment.

Eight (14.3%) additional patients with no gross evidence of disease had microscopic persistence in at lease one of the biopsies. In 5 of these patients, only 1 or 2 of the more than 20 biopsies were positive. Of the 8 patients, 5 had disease documented in the lymph nodes: 3 in pelvic nodes only, 1 patient had a positive periaortic lymph node, and 1 had both. In 3 of these patients, disease in the lymph nodes was the only positive finding. Cytology was positive in 4 patients, and in 2 it was the only positive finding. Peritoneal biopsies were positive in 3 patients, but were never the only positive biopsy site. Only a single diaphragm biopsy was positive (1 of 26, 3.8%), but this patient also had a positive peritoneal biopsy and cytology. The remaining 30 (53.6%) patients had macroscopic evidence of persistent cancer.

There were no operative deaths associated with the second-look procedure. Serious morbidity was seen in 4 patients (7.1%) and included postoperative pulmonary embolism, pneumonia, haemoperitoneum, and wound infection, all of which resolved without permanent sequelae.

Analysis of patient and clinical variables potentially related to outcome of the second-look laparotomy was performed. The variables significantly associated with a 'negative' observation were well and moderately differentiated tumours, the use of cisplatinum-containing combination chemotherapy, young patient age (<50 years), maximum residual tumour <0.5 cm in diameter remaining at the completion of the initial cytoreductive operation, and metastatic disease prior to cytoreduction of <10 cm in diameter. Variables not significantly associated with a negative second-look outcome included the maximum diameter of the primary tumour, the presence of ascites, and the number of cycles of chemotherapy.

Of the patients with metastatic tumours ranging from 1.5 to 10.0 cm who had residual tumour masses <1.5 cm in diameter following primary cytoreductive surgery, 36% had a negative second-look, while only 2 patients (15.4%) whose tumours were not optimally resected had a negative second-look. The overall percent negative second-look rate for optimal patients was 41.0% (16 out of 39), and 11.8% for non-optimal (2 of 17) (P <0.05). Both of these patients with non-optimal tumours were well differentiated and both patients received cisplatinum combination chemotherapy. Seven of 12 (58.7%) of the patients whose metastases were <1.5 cm in maximum diameter without requiring resection had a negative second-look. However, none of the 6 patients with >10 cm metastases had a negative second-look, regardless of the extent of tumour debulking performed.

The number of chemotherapy treatment cycles was related to the amount of residual disease and the probability of a negative second-look. There is no statistical difference in this sample between number of cycles of chemotherapy and the findings at second-look, in spite of the fact that the proportion of optimal patients treated with 6 to 9 cycles and 10 to 12 cycles of chemotherapy is less than those treated with >12 cycles. However, only 6 of 45 (13.3%) patients treated with the combination regimens received 12 cycles of chemotherapy, and this introduced a bias into this evaluation. Retrospectively, it was difficult to evaluate the precise reason why a given patient was treated with a specific number of chemotherapy cycles.

The five significant variables related to the probability of a negative second-look were entered into a multivariate discriminant analysis to determine which variables might properly classify the patients into either negative or positive second-look groups. Using this analysis, the primary tumour of well or moderate differentiation, the use of PAC (platinum, adriamycin, cyclophosphamide) chemotherapy, and small residual (<0.5 cm) maximum tumour diameter correctly classify a negative second-look in 12 of 18 patients and in 32 of 38 patients with positive second-looks. Thus, 44 of 56 (78.6%) patients were correctly classified in this sample.

Of the 15 patients who had a negative second-look after having received cisplatinum containing combination chemotherapy, 9 had residual tumours <0.5 cm, 4 had tumours 0.5–1.5 cm, and 2 had tumours ≥1.5 cm. Five of the 15 patients had grade 1 carcinomas, 9 were grade 2, and 1 was grade 3. Ten patients were ≤ 50 years old, and 5 were > 50 years.

Four of the 18 patients (33.3%) with negative second-look laparotomies have developed a recurrence of their cancer. The carcinomas recurred at 12, 15, 17 and 20 months (mean time to recurrence = 16 months) following the laparotomy. The remaining 14 patients have been followed for over 12 months so far. Recurrence was discovered in two patients in whom positive peritoneal cytology was documented at a third-look laparoscopy. Laparotomy performed on these patients revealed no gross evidence of disease. Two patients developed clinically apparent recurrences, one presenting with upper abdominal pain and a gastric mass and another with a pelvic mass. The former patient had an isolated recurrence in the gastric serosa, and the other in the pelvic cul-de-sac; each had all gross tumour resected. Three of these patients have received whole abdominal radiation therapy and are currently alive and clinically free of disease 12, 16 and 24 months post-treatment and one patient died 15 months later with liver metastases. The details of the subsequent management will be the subject of a separate report from our institution.

The median follow-up is 33 months. Of 18 patients who had a negative second-look laparotomy 17 (94.4%) are alive from 6 to 68 months from the time of laparotomy, compared with 5 of 8 (62.5%) patients with microscopic disease only who are alive at 12–42 months. The median survival for the 38 patients who had a positive second-look is 16.9 months. These patients are being followed and the clinical variables related to survival will be analysed when there has been sufficient follow-up.

Discussion

In the present study, we have confined our analysis to only those stage III patients who are clinically free of disease. The variables associated with a histopathologically negative second-look laparotomy in this group of patients were well and moderately differentiated tumour grade, the use of cisplatinum-containing combination chemotherapy, patient age ≤50 years, <0.5 cm maximum residual tumour after primary cytoreductive surgery, and ≤ 10 cm largest metastasis prior to cytoreduction. As determined by a discriminant analysis, a second-look is correctly classified in 78.6% of patients with low tumour grade, the use of cisplatinum containing combination chemotherapy, and small residual disease.

In previous reports in the literature, there has been inconsistency in the evaluation of data, since various definitions of second-look laparotomy have been employed. While some authors have restricted the definitions to those patients undergoing laparotomy who are clinically free of disease [4,5], others have included patients who have clinically appreciable evidence of progression [1–3,6,7]. An evaluation of clinical variables which might be associated with a negative second-look laparotomy has not been the principal subject of previous analyses.

In the present study, the rate of negative second-look operations was significantly greater for patients with grade 1 or 2 carcinomas compared with patients having grade 3 or 4 lesions. Previous reports have given conflicting data regarding the effect of tumour grade on the findings at second look [2,15], although several reports [1,3,4,6,7] have not specifically evaluated this variable.

Patients who received cisplatinum-containing combination chemotherapy had a significantly greater probability of a negative second-look compared with those patients who were treated with doxorubicin and cyclophosphamide (AC) combination therapy or with L-phenylalanine mustard (L-PAM). These data suggest that cisplatinum may have a significant impact in the treatment of epithelial malignancies and agree with previous reports which have indicated that cisplatinum chemotherapy in combination with other agents [13–17] possesses significant activity against advanced epithelial malignancies, compared with single agent therapies. Because most previous studies have utilised patients who received heterogeneous treatment, numbers have been insufficient to evaluate the influence of any particular type of therapy over another [3–7].

In this study, patients had a higher probability of a negative second-look if they received cisplatinum-containing chemotherapy than if they received AC or L-PAM, regardless of the histological grade.

With combination chemotherapy, the rate of negative second-look was the same for those patients who received 6 to 9 cycles of chemotherapy and those who received 10 to 12, which suggests that tumours that are responsive to therapy exhibit sensitivity early in their treatment. This is also true when the extent of residual disease is considered, i.e. the proportion of optimal patients did not influence outcome when corrected for the number of treatment cycles. Too few patients received less that 12 cycles of combination chemotherapy to assess the influence of more cycles of treatment on outcome. In this series, only 11 patients received L-PAM, but the use of >12 cycles of therapy in 5 of these patients produced only 1 patient with a negative second-look.

Since the tumour burden at the completion of the primary surgery is associated with outcome, the performance of optimal cytoreductive surgery in patients with metastases between 1.5 and 10.0 cm is probably an important variable relating to a pathological remission documented by second-look. These findings are in accord with our data regarding the influence of primary cytoreductive surgery on survival [10]. The amount of residual tumour at the completion of primary surgery is a strong predictor of outcome in several prior reports [2–5,7] and not significant in another [6]. However, the influence of cytoreduction per se in patients with metastatic disease in the findings at second-look has not been analysed.

Our data suggest the importance of a thorough operation for second-look. Since a significant proportion of patients without macroscopic tumour had their microscopic disease documented by 10% of the biopsies and cytologies taken, a large number of specimens must be submitted for evaluation. Indeed, since 5 of 26 (19.2%) patients without macroscopic disease had metastases detected in pelvic or periaortic lymph nodes, the performance of a thorough lymph node sampling is indicated in such patients. These data may in part explain the 30%–50% relapse rate reported in earlier series following purported negative second-look operations [1,2].

Based on our data, cisplatinum-containing combination chemotherapy appears to be a useful regimen with advanced stage epithelial ovarian malignancy. Using combination chemotherapy, shorter courses of chemotherapy—6 and 9 cycles of treatment—may induce as many remissions as longer courses of treatment, although this conclusion awaits longer follow-up and verification in prospective studies.

These data indicate that we cannot predict with certainty the outcome of second-look surgery on the basis of the analysis of clinical variables alone and, therefore, a surgical exploration in patients who are clinically free of disease is indicated until a more sensitive method is available for these patients. In order to standardise future analysis, we recommend that the term second-look should be reserved for an operation to evaluate tumour status only in those patients who are clinically free of disease following a prescribed course of chemotherapy.

References

1. Smith JP, Delgado G, Rutledge F (1976) Second-look operation in ovarian cancer. Cancer 38:1438–1442
2. Schwartz PE, Smith JP (1980) Second-look operation in ovarian cancer. Am J Obstet Gynecol 138:1124–1130
3. Phillips BD, Buchsbaum HJ, Lifshitz S (1979) Re-exploration after treatment for ovarian carcinoma. Gynecol Oncol 8:339–344
4. Curry SL, Zembo MM, Nahhas WA et al (1981) Second-look laparotomy for ovarian cancer. Gynecol Oncol 11:114–118
5. Webb MJ, Snyder JA, Williams TJ et al. (1982) Second-look laparotomy in ovarian cancer. Gynecol Oncol 14:285–293
6. Raju KS, McKinna JA, Barker GH et al. (1982) Second-look operations in the planned management of advanced ovarian carcinoma. Am J Obstet Gynecol 144:650–654
7. Roberts WS, Hodel K, Rich WM et al. (1982) Second-look laparotomy in the management of gynecologic malignancy. Gynecol Oncol 13:345–355
8. Greco FA, Julian CG, Richardson RL et al (1981) Advanced ovarian cancer: brief intensive combination chemotherapy and second-look operation. Obstet Gynecol 58:199–204
9. Allen MS, Hertig AT (1949) Carcinoma of the ovary. Am J Obstet Gynecol 58:640–655
10. Hacker NF, Berek JS, Lagasse LD et al. (1983) Primary cytoreductive surgery for epithelial ovarian cancer. Obstet Gynecol 61:413–420
11. Berek JS, Hacker NF, Lagasse LD et al. (1983) Survival of patients following secondary cytoreductive surgery in ovarian cancer. Obstet Gynecol 61:189–193
12. Dixon WJ (1981) BMDP statistical software. UCLA Press, Berkeley, California, pp 519–537
13. Bruckner HW, Cohen CJ, Goldberg JD et al. (1981) Improved chemotherapy for ovarian cancer with cis-diamminedichloroplatinum and adriamycin. Cancer 47:2288–2295
14. Williams CJ, Mead B, Arnold A et al. (1982) Chemotherapy of advanced ovarian carcinoma: initial experience using a platinum-based combination. Cancer 49:1778–1783
15. Bruckner HW, Cohen CJ, Goldberg JD et al. (1983) Cisplatin regimens and improved prognosis of patients with poorly differentiated ovarian cancer. Am J Obstet Gynecol 145:653–658
16. Ehrlich CE, Einhorn L, Williams SD et al. (1979) Chemotherapy for stage III-IV epithelial ovarian cancer with cis-dichlorodiammineplatinum (II), adriamycin, and cyclophosphamide: A preliminary report. CA Treat Rep 63:281–288
17. Decker DG, Fleming TR, Malkasian GD et al. (1982) Cyclophosphamide plus cis-platinum in combination: Treatment program for stage III or IV ovarian carcinoma. Obstet Gynecol 40:481–487

20 · Second-look Surgery in Ovarian Cancer— Some Reservations

G.E. Smart and D.I.M. Farquharson

Introduction

Wangensteen in 1949 was the first to advocate the use of second-look surgery in patients with cancer of the bowel in an attempt to improve survival by detecting, and if necessary removing, residual tumour at six monthly intervals [1]. Since then gynaecologists have, with varying degrees of enthusiasm, come to accept it as a part of the optimal management of patients with epithelial ovarian cancer. It is being increasingly advocated to assess disease status after chemotherapy, not only to enable further debulking to be accomplished and for changes in therapy to be instituted but, where negative, to allow chemotherapy to be stopped altogether [2,3,4].

Schwartz and Smith, for example, strongly support the value of second-look surgery to allow further debulking of tumour. Their survival curves, reproduced in Fig. 20.1, suggest that debulking down to less than 2 cm deposits at second-look offers, with additional chemotherapy, the same 30% 5-year survival rate as total removal of tumour, in advanced disease [5]. It is interesting, however, to note that unresectable tumour allowing biopsy only, carries a better prognosis than either of these two groups for up to $2\frac{1}{2}$ years after second-look surgery, and no information is provided about the histological grade of the tumours in each group, which in itself may well be the factor that is more contributory to survival than the operation itself.

Although the principle of second-look surgery has therefore been accepted in most oncological circles, we still lack convincing evidence from adequate controls as to its true worth, and have continually to remind ourselves of the disadvantages as well as the benefits of the procedure [4]. Whilst survival rates for advanced

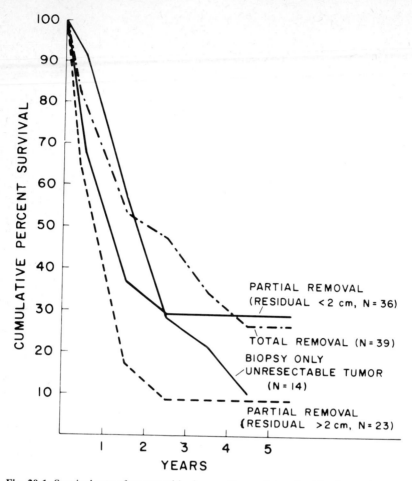

Fig. 20.1. Survival rate after second-look operation as determined by the maximum diameter of the largest residual tumour mass upon completion of the operation. (Schwartz [3]; reproduced by kind permission of the author and the Editor of *Clinics in Obstetrics and Gynaecology*).

cancer of the ovary remain low in spite of new and exciting chemotherapeutic combinations, it behoves us to question whether the possible benefits offered by second-look surgery in terms of increased survival or cure for some, are justified by the inconvenience, psychological trauma and possible increased morbidity and decreased quality of survival of others.

Background

In this study we have reviewed two groups of patients with epithelial cancer of the ovary referred to the Combined Gynaecological Oncology Clinic at the

Edinburgh Royal Infirmary, the first group from January 1976 to August 1980 and the second from September 1980 to December 1982. Each group has been sub-divided into two sub-groups according to whether, at initial operation, there was no obvious residual disease remaining (so-called Protocol I disease) or whether there was macroscopic intra-abdominal disease left (so-called Protocol III). Patients with residual pelvic disease only (so-called Protocol II) have not been considered as their numbers at the time of this analysis were too small. In 1980 our treatment was standardised so that patients with Protocol I disease are now randomised between no additional therapy or whole abdominal radiation and pelvic booster (following the Toronto practice), and patients with Protocol III disease randomised between a single alkylating agent (prednimustine) or quad-ruple therapy (prednimustine, cisplatinum, 5-fluorouracil and hexa-methylmelamine) [6]. Prior to 1980 the management in both Protocol I and III groups was much less standardised following initial surgery but usually consisted of single alkylating agent chemotherapy in the form of chlorambucil, followed by a cyclical regime of chlorambucil, methotrexate and 5-fluorouracil (CMF) or treosulphan, chlorambucil and prednisolone (TCP), with occasionally Adriamycin added in patients with non-responsive disease. In the first group of patients (i.e. prior to 1980) second-look laparotomy was frequently but not always performed (at a mean time of 18 months after initial surgery in Protocol I disease and 13 months in Protocol III disease), whilst in the second (1980–82) group the treatment protocol included second-look surgery after 12 months in Protocol I (mean time of 13 months) and after 6 courses of chemotherapy in Protocol III disease (mean time 8.7 months). The second-look procedure was carried out either by the original referring consultant or one of two gynaecologists with a special interest in gynaecological oncology.

This preliminary study compares the crude survival rates of both main groups of patients (pre-1980 and post-1980) and then proceeds to analyse those second-look procedures in the post-1980 group, with the intention of determining the value of the procedure from the point of view of diagnosis and treatment of residual disease. We are not concerned in this paper with the comparison of different methods of chemotherapy or radiotherapy but are merely concerned with report-ing our experience of second-look laparotomy in these two main groups of ovarian cancer, with the intention of evaluating its contribution towards patient management.

Characteristics of Groups Studied

Table 20.1 shows that there were 128 patients in the 'historical' group (pre-1980) and 64 patients in the trial group with Protocol I, II and III disease following initial laparotomy. Of these, 40 with Protocol I or III disease had second-look laparotomies in the historical group, compared with 30 in the trial group, but only 23 of the latter have been followed up sufficiently long for a 15 month survival curve to be drawn.

Breakdown of the material into individual cell types shows that the two groups are very similar apart from an apparent under-representation of serous and over-

Table 20.1. Numbers of patients in pre-trial and trial groups (the 30 patients in the trial group having second-look laparotomies include one patient with Protocol II disease)

	Pre-trial January 1966 – August 1980	Trial September 1980 – December 1982
n	128	64
2nd looks	40	30
2nd looks (15 months follow-up)	40	23

representation of unspecified-origin tumours in the historical group (see Table 20.2). However, subsequent re-examination of the older histological material (of which only approximately two-thirds was available for analysis) shows that many of this latter group were in fact serous type, and thus the two groups are even more comparable. The distribution of histological grades within each tumour 'group' is seen in Fig. 20.2. The histogram shows that for Protocol III tumours the distribution of grades is virtually identical for both historical and trial groups, although for the trial patients in Protocol I there is an under-representation of well differentiated and over-representation of moderately differentiated lesions relative to the historical group. On the evidence, however, of several workers, including a multivariate analysis from Sigurdsson and colleagues in Sweden, the well and the moderately differentiated tumours behave similarly with respect to outcome as distinct from the poorly differentiated tumours, which have a much poorer prognosis [7]. If, therefore, the well and moderately differentiated groups are considered together, there is very little difference between the historical and trial groups. This relationship between cell grade and outcome in our own patients is seen in Figs. 20.3 and 20.4 and will be referred to again later.

Survival Rates

Figure 20.3 shows 20-month survival curves for a total of 106 patients in the pre-trial group (i.e. pre-1980) compared with curves for a total of 44 patients in the trial group (i.e. post-1980). These curves include all patients, with and without

Table 20.2. Comparison between tumour histology of pre-trial and trial groups

	Pre-trial January 1966 – August 1980	Trial September 1980 – December 1982
n	128	64
Histology		
Serous	29.8	51.6
Mucinous	15.8	15.6
Endometrioid	19.3	15.6
Clear cell	10.5	6.3
Mixed	3.5	3.1
Unspecified	21.0	7.8

CORRELATION BETWEEN TUMOUR GRADE
AND TUMOUR STAGE

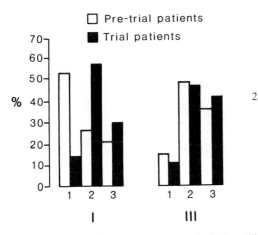

Fig. 20.2. Correlation between tumour grade (1, 2 and 3) and tumour stage (normally early, Protocol I disease, and late, Protocol III disease).

SURVIVAL FROM TIME OF PRESENTATION PROTOCOLS I AND III

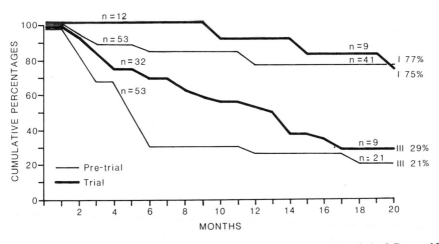

Fig. 20.3. Twenty-month survival curves for both pre-trial and trial patients in both Protocol I and III groups, from time of presentation at 0.

second-look surgery. It can be seen that within each protocol there is no significant difference (confirmed on chi-squared testing) between the 20-month survival rates of the historical group compared with the trial group of patients. Although there is a suggestion of a significant slowing of death rate in the early months in the trial patients with Protocol III disease, this has deliberately not been confirmed by log rank analysis as it would be dangerous to draw further conclusions from such

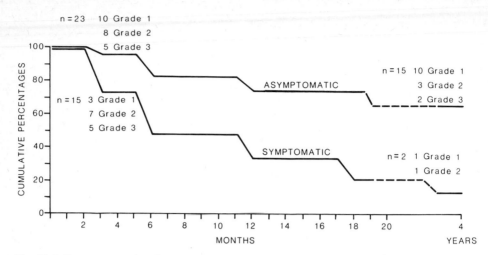

Fig. 20.4. Curves comparing the outcome of symptomatic with asymptomatic pre-trial patients from the time of second-look surgery at point 0. Both groups contain patients with both Protocol I and Protocol III disease, and show the favourable effect of tumour grade on survival.

raw data, as not only have different proportions within each group been treated completely differently in terms of chemotherapy, but also unequal proportions have been subjected to second-look procedures at different times after initial surgery. Moreover in the historical group the decision to perform a second-look procedure will have varied considerably from consultant to consultant depending on his/her personal views as well as the condition of the patient, whereas in the trial group a second-look laparotomy is included in the protocol as described previously. The very most we are entitled to conclude from the 20-month survival data is that there is no evidence that a more rigid chemotherapeutic protocol together with a routine second-look laparotomy (on those patients who survived long enough) is any better than less standardised chemotherapy with no 'built-in' provision for a routine second-look procedure.

Prognostic Variables

If we now compare the outcome of those patients who were asymptomatic prior to second-look surgery (that is those who had absolutely no clinical evidence of disease) with the outcome of those who were symptomatic we see an obvious and not entirely unexpected survival pattern (see Figs. 20.4 and 20.5). We also see that the survivors are composed of a much higher proportion of patients with well differentiated tumours. The vast majority of deaths had occurred in those patients with poorly differentiated tumours, and most of those with well differentiated

2nd LOOK SURGERY SURVIVAL CURVES FOR PATIENTS IN TRIAL 1980-1982

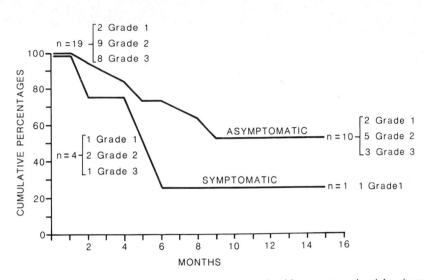

Fig. 20.5. Curves comparing the outcome of symptomatic with asymptomatic trial patients from the time of second-look surgery at point 0. Both groups contain patients with both Protocol I and Protocol III disease, and show the favourable effect of tumour grade on survival.

growths have survived. One is tempted to wonder whether survival after second-look surgery may be related more to inherent tumour behaviour than to any effect of surgery itself.

Another prognostic indicator has been shown by several workers to be the size of residual tumour mass after primary surgery [5,8,9,10]. We have looked at this variable on outcome in the trial patients and find that the size of residual tumour mass bears a direct relationship to the tumour status discovered at second-look laparotomy, which in turn has a direct bearing on prognosis. Thus all the patients who were thought to be tumour-free at second-look laparotomy were all alive at 15 months, whilst the outcome for those with a positive second-look operation is predictably poor (Table 20.3). The tumour status at second-look surgery is a good predictor of survival and up to 15 months after the procedure only one of the ten patients with negative second-look laparotomies has turned up with recurrent tumour. This 10% figure compares with other reports of between 4.8 and 17.6% [5,8,10,11].

Table 20.3. Relationship between residual tumour after primary surgery, findings at second-look procedure and outcome at 15 months

Number	1st operation residual tumour	2nd look tumour free	2nd look residual tumour
11	0	6 (all alive)	5 (3 dead)
10	<2 cm	3 (all alive)	7 (3 dead)
9	>2 cm	1 (all alive)	8 (6 dead)

Complications of Second-Look Surgery

Our major complication rate following second-look surgery has remained fairly constant over the years of this study (Table 20.4). Major complications have included severe wound infection, complete wound dehiscence, uraemia, confusional state, incisional hernia, paralytic ileus, pulmonary embolus, and a fatal cerebrovascular accident, giving a major complication rate of 26% in the historical group and 23% in the trial group. These figures compare with a major complication rate of 23% calculated from Schwartz and Smith's recently published data [5]. Several workers have suggested laparoscopy as an alternative to laparotomy in an attempt to avoid this sort of complication rate [12,13,14,15,16,17]. Berek initially reported a major complication rate from laparoscopy of 14% (all requiring laparotomy, mainly due to small bowel perforation) but following the introduction of a small gauge needlescope in order to select a safer site for laparoscopic insertion, he reduced this rate to 1.2% [18]. Rosenoff, [14], Smith [15], Quinn [12] and Piver [13] are some of the many who have advocated second-look laparoscopy in patients in complete clinical remission. Piver and colleagues take washings at the time of second-look laparoscopy from the pelvis and paracolic spaces, and submit them for immediate frozen section analysis, a process which takes 30 min or so whilst the patient is still under general anaesthesia. Positive laparoscopy including cytology can spare up to 40% of patients a more extensive surgical procedure with fewer major complications, but to date the view is that cytology has too high a false negative rate, and a negative laparoscopy with cytology therefore should be followed by a formal laparotomy [2,13]. Our own experience, although limited, in non-trial patients does suggest that it is a safe procedure and one which should possibly be considered for use in the follow-up of so-called asymptomatic Protocol III patients where the chances of residual disease not being amenable to therapy are so much more likely.

Analysis of Second-Look Laparotomies (post-1980)

Diagnostic Value

We have reviewed the records of the patients in the trial who have had second-look surgery in an attempt to determine its diagnostic value.

Protocol I Disease

Table 20.5 shows that of the 11 patients who had second-look laparotomies in Protocol I disease, 6 had negative findings and were alive and asymptomatic at 15 months follow-up. All these 6 were asymptomatic pre-operatively and it seems

Table 20.4. Major complications of second-look surgery

Trial	7/30	23%	Severe wound infection
			Wound dehiscence (2)
			Perforated bowel
			Uraemia
			Paralytic ileus (2)
Pre-trial	10/38	26%	Severe wound infection (2)
			Wound dehiscence (4)
			Incisional hernia
			Pulmonary embolism
			Confusional state
			CVA (death)

from this experience that this information could have been achieved by cytology of peritoneal washings alone without necessitating laparotomy (although admittedly one patient did not have washings taken).

Of these 11 patients, 5 had positive findings at second-look laparotomy of whom 4 were found to have gross intraperitoneal disease and 1 nodal disease only. Two, including the 1 with nodal disease, were still alive at 15 months and both these were asymptomatic prior to surgery. The patient with nodal disease had false negative cytology of peritoneal washings.

It would seem therefore that of the 11 patients with Protocol I disease, cytology alone would have missed only 1 positive and correctly diagnosed the remaining 10 cases.

Protocol III Disease

In Protocol III disease, 18 patients had second-look laparotomy, of whom only 3 were negative, and were still alive, and 15 positive, of whom 6 were alive at 15 months. If we look more closely at these groups we find that of the 3 negatives, 2 had adequate laparotomies (although without lymph node biopsies) with negative cytology, but the third had what can only be considered inadequate surgery because of widespread adhesions, and no peritoneal washings being obtained. The 15 positive cases all had gross residual disease and of those who had peritoneal washings, all were positive.

From this information, it would again seem that cytology alone would probably have provided similar information to laparotomy, with no complications.

Table 20.5. Outcome, at 15 months, related to findings at second-look laparotomy

	Protocol I	Protocol III
n	11	18
Negative	6 (6 alive)	3 (3 alive)
Positive	5 (2 alive)	15 (6 alive)
	(3 dead)	

Therapeutic Value

Protocol I Disease

As far as the Protocol I patients are concerned, with the exception of the patient with nodal disease, all those with positive findings had biopsies only, none being suitable for debulking, and therefore no obvious therapeutic benefit accrued from the operation itself.

Protocol III Disease

Of the 15 positive second-looks in Protocol III disease, debulking was impossible in 11, and of the remaining 4 in whom it was possible to debulk to less than 2 cm deposits of residual tumour, 3 have subsequently died within 8 months of surgery, and the remaining one is still alive although deteriorating rapidly. Five of the positive second-look patients have subsequently died at between 9 and 25 months. It is hard to escape the conclusion that therapeutic gains were virtually nil as second-look surgery has benefited at the most only one patient.

Peritoneal Lavage

In an attempt to provide the same diagnostic information as second-look surgery with regard to the presence or absence of residual tumour, we have recently carried out a pilot study on peritoneal lavage the day before proposed second-look surgery. This involves the introduction of 2 litres of normal saline into the peritoneal cavity under local anaethesia. Thirty minutes later the saline is drained away and sent off for immediate cytology. Of the first 28 patients so far studied, 5 false negative results have been obtained, 2 patients having positive retro-peritoneal lymph nodes as the only evidence of residual disease. Correlation has been good except where there have been solitary nodules in the presence of extensive intra-abdominal adhesions preventing adequate circulation of the lavage fluid. No significant morbidity has been encountered. (J.R.B. Livingstone and M. McIntyre 1983, personal communication). This study is being continued.

Discussion and Conclusions

This paper questions the role of second-look surgery in patient management in the light of recent Edinburgh experience. It does not set out to compare different modalities of treatment of cancer of the ovary. Whilst we have confirmed the importance with respect to survival of tumour grade and residual tumour mass following primary surgery, we have not found second-look laparotomy, as currently performed, to be of much value in terms of either diagnosis or therapy. We question whether previous evidence supporting the value of further debulking at second-look laparotomy may not be related more to initial residual tumour mass and grade rather than to the secondary procedure itself, and we feel that it is far from being established that second-look procedures add to the length or quality of survival of patients with ovarian cancer.

These doubts are certainly strengthened by our own analysis, admittedly in a small number of patients so far, in whom therapeutic advantages seem to be almost nil. There is a real danger that with the aim of helping the few, relatively major but often inadequate procedures would be carried out on the many. Quite apart from the well-being of the latter not being improved, their remaining months may actually be rendered even more distressing than would otherwise have been the case.

As far as the diagnostic value of second-look surgery is concerned, it would seem from our own experience that unless the surgeon is prepared to carry out a thorough sampling of pelvic and para-aortic lymph nodes, then the practice of second-look laparotomy is hard to justify, and any diagnostic information would probably be more conveniently available by cytology alone with virtual absence of morbidity. Such a relatively non-invasive approach would admittedly have a certain false negative rate (probably little higher than laparotomy itself when not combined with lymphadenectomy) and it would certainly not allow for quantitative estimates of residual disease to be made in order to assess the degree of response to radiation or chemotherapy. Nevertheless, we question whether the gains in diagnostic information for relatively few patients can justify such invasive procedures being performed on the many. As ultrasonography and computerised tomography are of only limited value as aids to the diagnosis of residual ovarian cancer [19], it is probable that in the future our diagnostic energies should be directed more towards the use of cytology combined with more sophisticated tumour localisation techniques, such as NMR and immunoscintigraphy using radiolabelled monoclonal tumour antibodies (E.M. Symonds 1983, personal communication, and [20]), and that these and other relatively non-invasive methods may well render second-look surgery for diagnosis an obsolete procedure.

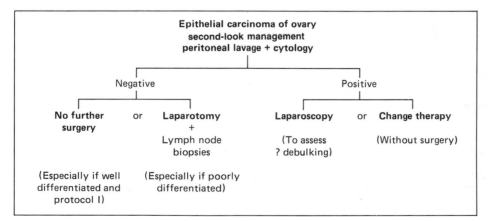

Fig. 20.6. Suggested scheme for second-look management dependent on results of peritoneal cytology.

Until such techniques are developed we would advise that where possible second-look surgery be carried out only in the context of properly controlled clinical trials, so that maximum information regarding its efficacy may be obtained. We would also tentatively suggest that a scheme such as that outlined in Fig. 20.6 should be used on which to base the management of patients with ovarian cancer. This scheme would not only allow us to treat patients who are already unfit physically and psychologically without resorting to laparotomy in many instances, but could also be used as a basis for randomisation between 'surgery' and 'no surgery' to provide the true control groups that are necessary in order to evaluate the real value of second-look laparotomy or laparoscopy in the management of patients with ovarian cancer.

References

1. Wangensteen OH (1949) Cancer of colon and rectum. Wis Med J 48:591–597
2. Piver MS (1983) In: Singer A and Jordan J (eds) Ovarian malignancies. Current Reviews in Obstetrics and Gynaecology, 4. Churchill Livingstone, Edinburgh, p 116
3. Schwartz PE (1983) Current status of the second-look operation in ovarian cancer. Clin Obstet Gynaecol 10:245–259
4. Smart GE, Farquharson DIM (1985) In: Hudson CR (ed) Ovarian cancer. Oxford University Press, pp 323–333
5. Schwartz PE, Smith JP (1980) Second-look operations in ovarian cancer. Am J Obstet Gynecol 138:1124–1130
6. The Edinburgh Ovarian Cancer Trial Co-ordinators, Smyth J, Ludgate S, Livingstone JRB, Smart GE
7. Sigurdsson K, Alm P, Gullberg B, Johnsson JE, Trope C (1984) Stadiumindelning och differentieringsgrad faktorer som paverkar overlevnaden vid ovarialcancer. Lakartidningen 81:2354–2357
8. Curry SL, Zembo MM, Wahhas WA et al. (1981) Second-look laparotomy for ovarian cancer. Gynec Oncol 11:114-118
9. Wharton JT, Herson J (1981) Surgery for common epithelial tumours of the ovary. Cancer 48:582–589
10. Greco FA, Julian CG, Richardson RL et al. (1981) Advanced ovarian cancer: Brief intensive combination chemotherapy and second-look operation. Obstet Gynecol 58:199–205
11. Phillips BP, Buchsbaum HJ, Lifschitz S (1979) Re-exploration after treatment for ovarian cancer. Gynecol Oncol 8:339–345
12. Quinn MA, Bishop GJ, Campbell JJ et al. (1980) Laparoscopic follow-up of patients with ovarian carcinoma. Br J Obstet Gynaecol 87:1132–1139
13. Piver MS, Lele SB, Barlow JJ et al. (1980) Second-look laparotomy prior to proposed second-look laparotomy. Obstet Gynecol 55:571–573
14. Rosenoff SH, DeVita T Jr, Hubbard S et al. (1977) Peritoneoscopy in the staging and follow-up of ovarian cancer. Semin Oncol 2:223-228
15. Smith WG, Day TG Jr, Smith JP (1977) The use of laparoscopy to determine the results of chemotherapy for ovarian cancer. J Reprod Med 18: 259–560
16. Barker GH (1983) Chemotherapy of gynaecological malignancies. Castle House Publications, London, p 78
17. Ozols RF, Fisher RI, Anderson T et al. (1981) Peritoneoscopy in the staging and follow-up of ovarian cancer. Am J Obstet Gynecol 140:611–619
18. Berek JS, Griffiths CT, Leventhall JM (1981) Laparoscopy for second-look evaluation in ovarian cancer. Obstet Gynecol 58:192–198
19. Kerr-Wilson RHJ, Shingleton HM, Orr JW et al. (1984) The use of ultrasound and computed tomography screening in the management of gynecologic cancer patients. Gynecol Oncology 18:54–61
20. Johnson IR, Symonds EM, Worthington BS et al. (1984) Imaging ovarian tumours by nuclear magnetic resonance. Br J Obstet Gynaecol 91:260–264

21 · A Decision Theory Analysis of Radiotherapeutic and Chemotherapeutic Toxicity in the Management of Ovarian Cancer

R.A. Potish and L.B. Twiggs

Introduction

Many decisions in the management of cancer contain a component of uncertainty. A treatment which benefits one patient may harm another patient. An 'average' response to therapy is only occasionally observed: some patients respond surprisingly well, while others fare unexpectedly poorly. A particularly frustrating manifestation of these elements of probability is the apparent randomness of therapeutic successes and failures in patients who appear to be closely matched for all known prognostic factors.

This indeterminacy permeates the management of epithelial carcinoma of the ovary. Although both ionising radiation and alkylating agents can cure some women, overall survival has remained unsatisfactory. Both retrospective reviews and prospective trials have obtained conflicting data concerning the relative efficacy of these modalities. In addition, either therapy can engender morbidity and mortality. Although multiagent chemotherapy offers the hope of greater survival rates, it also raises the spectre of increased iatrogenic toxicity.

The patient and physician thus face difficult choices in attempting to select the optimal therapy. The possible benefit of treatment is cure of cancer. Risks range from failure to cure by selection of ineffective therapy to severe enteric damage from radiotherapy and leukaemia from chemotherapy. The best treatment 'on the average' may not be the best treatment for an individual patient. The present study will demonstrate methods of minimising treatment-related toxicity for individual patients. Although models will be shown for alkylating agents and radiotherapy, the principles of this analysis can be applied throughout the field of oncology.

Materials and Methods

In order to establish the toxicity of abdominal–pelvic radiation therapy, three series were employed (Table 21.1) [1–3]. Severe enteric morbidity, manifest primarily by small bowel obstruction, occurred in 6.3% of the 349 patients. Four fatal complications ensued, yielding a rate of 1.1%. Three deaths were secondary to enteric injury and one secondary to hepatic damage, although it was questionable whether radiation actually caused two of these four deaths [1]. Both the Princess Margaret Hospital (PMH) and the M.D. Anderson Hospital and Tumor Institute (MDAH) used the moving strip technique, while the University of Minnesota Hospitals (UMH) used an open field technique. The PMH delivered 2250 cGy (rad) in 10 fractions to the pelvis followed by 2250 cGy in 10 fractions to the abdominal strips, while the MDAH abdominal strip dose was 2600 to 2800 cGy in 12 fractions, with an additional 2000 cGy in 10 fractions given to the pelvis either before or after the abdominal therapy. The UMH technique administered 2000 cGy in 20 fractions to the abdominal fields followed by 2975 cGy in 17 fractions to the pelvis.

The 111 UMH patients were analysed in detail to generate logistic models to predict chronic enteric damage. Operative intervention was required in 7 patients with small bowel obstruction, and 2 of these subsequently developed fistulae. Preliminary analysis and further details have already been published [3]. The current study used the Cox logistic method to predict enteric injury as a function of physique and prior surgery to individual patients [4].

For computation of the probability of alkylating agent-associated leukaemia, the data from a study of five randomised clinical trials were used [5]. The cumulative risk of acute non-lymphocytic leukaemia was 13.2% in patients receiving Alkeran and 9.6% in patients receiving any alkylating agent. Of 10 women developing leukaemia after Alkeran, 9 had received greater than 700 mg. The MDAH data were used to calculate leukaemia rates relative to initial chemotherapy dose. While no patient initially receiving less than 700 mg of Alkeran developed leukaemia, 9.5% (4 of 42) receiving a greater initial dose did develop leukaemia [5]. As 63% of patients survived long-term disease-free, the incidence of leukaemia was 15.9% [6]. This rate must be regarded as only approximate as

Table 21.1. Probabilities of radiation-related morbidity and mortality

Institution	Enteric injury	Death
UMH	0.063 (7/111)	0.000 (0/111)
MDAH (2)	0.126 (11/87)	0.023 (2/87)
PMH (1)	0.026 (4/151)	0.013 (2/151)
Total	0.063 (22/349)	0.011 (4/349)

the patients who received greater initial doses may have had different probabilities of survival. However, the MDAH rate is compatible with a study from the Radiumhemmet which found a 33% leukaemia incidence in patients receiving 800 mg or more of Alkeran and a zero incidence in patients receiving less than 800 mg [7].

The tools of decision theory offered a means of quantifying the optimal choice of treatment. For this analysis, it was necessary to assign numerical values to the outcomes of enteric injury and leukaemia. Standard statistical terminology designates these values as costs or losses [8]. A fatal complication was arbitrarily assigned a cost of one hundred, while an absence of complication had a cost of zero. A non-fatal bowel injury would in turn be given a cost intermediate between zero and one hundred. The expected cost was obtained by multiplying the value of the individual cost or loss by its probability of occurrence [8].

Results

The logistic model predicted complications by using the equations:
$$P = 1 / (1 + \exp(F))$$
$$F = A + Bx + Cy$$
where P was the probability of small bowel obstruction, exp was the natural exponent, x was the number of pelvic and abdominal operations, and y was the prescription depth in centimetres of abdominal portal, used as an index of physique [3]. A, B, and C were constants estimated from the 111 patients. Separate models were created for the entire group of patients and for the long-term survivors. Figure 21.1 shows the probability of small bowel obstruction monotonically falling with increasing index of physique. This probability was

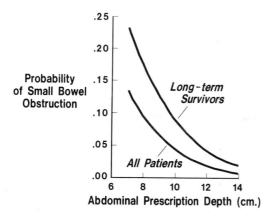

Fig. 21.1. The probability of small bowel obstruction is presented as a function of body physique. The abdominal prescription depth of the radiation portals has been used as an index of physique. The complication probability is greatest in thin women and is higher in long-term survivors than in the overall group.

Table 21.2. Probabilities of radiation-related small bowel obstruction as a function of prior surgery

Number of surgeries	All patients	Long-term survivors only
1	0.03	0.05
2	0.06	0.11
3	0.11	0.21
4	0.21	0.38
5	0.35	0.59
6	0.53	0.76

greater in the long-term survivors than in the entire group. Table 21.2 presents complication probabilities as a function of prior surgery.

When number of operations (x) and abdominal thickness (y) in centimetres are combined in a logistic model, F equals $-3.384 -1.019x +0.92y$ for the entire group of patients and $-3.474 -1.027x +0.85y$ for the long-term survivors. In order to predict complication probabilities with these two variables, F is substituted into the above logistic equation. A typical patient, with two previous operations and a prescribed treatment depth of 10 cm, would have a 0.05 complication probability if she were a long-term survivor. On the other hand, a woman with three prior surgeries and a depth of 8 cm would have an enteric injury probability of 0.44, while a woman with one operation and a depth of 12 cm would have only a 0.003 chance of bowel damage. In order to measure the accuracy of the model, Table 21.3 presents standard deviations at various predicted probabilities.

Figure 21.2 schematically portrays a dose–response relation for the induction of acute non-lymphocytic leukaemia by Alkeran. The MDAH and Radiumhemmet data are presented by the horizontal lines, and it is hypothesised that there is a very small risk of leukaemia at very low doses of Alkeran. However, there are insufficient data to depict accurately the point at which the incidence of leukaemia starts to rise. The point at which the incidence of leukaemia plateaus is also unknown.

Figure 21.3 demonstrates the effect of cancer mortality on the incidence of treatment-related deaths. Leukaemia occurred in 13% of long-term survivors exposed to Alkeran, whilst 2% of the long-term survivors receiving radiation therapy eventually died from complications. As the proportion of deaths from cancer increases, iatrogenic deaths decline proportionally.

Table 21.3. Standard deviations for predicted complication probabilities with logistic model with both physique and surgery for long-term survivors

Predicted probability	Standard deviation of predicted probability
0.75	0.25
0.58	0.21
0.30	0.16
0.22	0.10
0.13	0.09
0.06	0.04
0.03	0.02
0.00	0.01

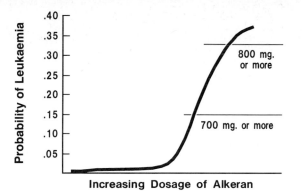

Fig. 21.2. The probability of acute non-lymphocytic leukaemia is presented as a function of increasing dosage of Alkeran. The lower horizontal line represents the M. D. Anderson Hospital leukaemia incidence in patients receiving 700 m or more of Alkeran [5, 6]. The higher horizontal line depicts the Radiumhemmet leukaemia incidence in patients receiving 800 mg of Alkeran or more [7]. A hypothetical dose–response curve is drawn through these ranges. It is hypothesised that there is a small leukaemia risk at low doses of Alkeran. The point at which the leukaemia incidence plateaus at high doses of Alkeran is unknown.

Probability of Mortality in Ovarian Cancer

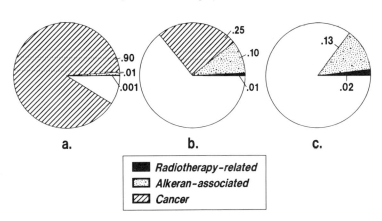

Fig. 21.3. The three circle graphs symbolise patterns of mortality probabilities from cancer and from therapy. If as many as 0.90 of women die from cancer **a**, only 0.001 would have radiation-related mortality and 0.01 would have Alkeran-associated mortality. If fewer women die from cancer, iatrogenic mortality rates will be higher among the long-term survivors **b**. In the extreme case **c** of no cancer deaths, 0.02 of patients receiving radiation and 0.13 of patients receiving Alkeran may die from late effects of therapy.

   The decision theory analysis is shown in Figs. 21.4 and 21.5. Acute non-lymphocytic leukaemia developing after alkylating agent therapy is almost invariably fatal, and this is assigned a reference or baseline cost of 100. Three deaths occurred among the 22 patients developing severe enteric injury after radiation, giving a mortality rate of 14%. Thus, if mortality were the only concern, Fig. 21.4 should be used, with a cost of 100 for haematopoietic toxicity and a cost of 14 for

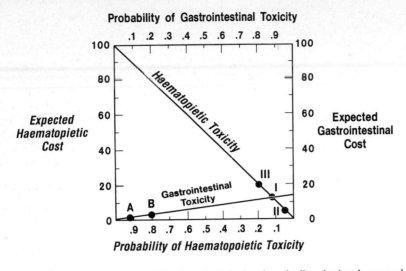

Fig. 21.4. The expected cost of leukaemia is depicted on the line sloping downward from left to right. The expected cost of enteric injury is depicted on the line sloping upward from left to right. The cost of leukaemia is 100 and the cost of enteric injury is 14, corresponding to their respective mortality rates. Costs are displayed vertically and probabilities are displayed horizontally. See text for additional explanation.

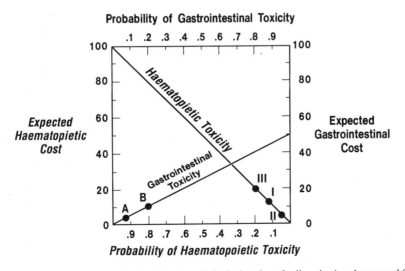

Fig. 21.5. The expected cost of leukaemia is depicted on the line sloping downward from left to right. The expected cost of enteric injury is depicted on the line sloping upward from left to right. The cost of leukaemia is 100 and the cost of enteric injury is 50. The enteric cost is assigned a greater value than in Fig. 21.4 in order to take morbidity in account. Costs are displayed vertically and probabilities are displayed horizontally. See text for additional explanation.

gastrointestinal toxicity. However, patients with non-fatal severe chronic enteric morbidity also incur substantial cost. If this cost is added to the mortality, then an enteric cost of 50 (Fig. 21.5) may be more representative. Although these costs are arbitrary, the patient and physician are free to assign any other costs.

Figures 21.4 and 21.5 may be used to obtain the expected cost by multiplying the complication cost by its corresponding probability. The probabilities are placed on the horizontal axes in opposite directions for ease of presentation. In order to ascertain the expected cost at a given probability, simply place a perpendicular line at the appropriate probability until it intersects the relevant line. As an example, point III on Figs. 21.4 and 21.5 corresponds to an expected cost of 20 for leukaemia at a probability of 0.20. Point A, at an enteric probability of 0.08, yields an expected cost of 1 on Fig. 21.4, and 4 on Fig. 21.5. Both figures have identical leukaemia costs, but Fig. 21.5 has a greater enteric cost because it takes morbidity as well as mortality into account.

The expected enteric cost at point B may be greater or less than the expected leukaemic cost at point II, depending on the assumed values of the complications. As shown by points A and B and I through III, expected cost increases linearly with complication incidence.

Discussion

Decision theory formalises many intuitive concerns of patients and physicians. Particularly relevant is the concept of a hierarchy of valued outcomes. In general, cure of cancer is the paramount objective of the oncologist. However, the therapeutic modalities employed against cancer can cause substantial morbidity and mortality. In addition, there are a host of other potentially important values, ranging from emotions to finances. Despite its obvious importance, the enumeration of these values is not an easy task.

As cancer therapy becomes more effective, more patients survive long enough to develop serious complications. The 13% cumulative incidence of acute non-lymphocytic leukaemia in women exposed to Alkeran furnishes an important example of this phenomenon. There is an analagous, though lesser, rate of severe enteric injury from radiotherapy. Figure 21.3 demonstrates the extent to which recurrent cancer conceals iatrogenic mortality. When advanced ovarian cancer is treated, the 5%–10% cure rate will allow very few late complications to be expressed [9]. However, as the cure rate rises, the complication rate will increase proportionally. A treatment programme which includes both an alkylating agent and radiation will lead to both leukaemia and enteric injury if enough patients survive for a long enough time [10]. The importance of severe late complications will be greatest when adjuvant therapy of uncertain efficacy is administered to patients with relatively good prognoses.

If cure of cancer is the major goal, then treatment can be chosen on that criterion alone. However, even if that is done, as many as 15% of patients who are cured may die from the treatment. If cure rates are similar with radiation and alkylating agents, then choice of therapy can be dictated by minimising toxicity. Two prospective randomised clinical trials found no substantial difference between these two modalities, while a third found radiation to be superior

[1,2,11]. This issue may never be resolved as it has been replaced by another controversy between single-agent and multiagent chemotherapy [12].

Assuming that cure rates are equivalent for at least some subsets of patients, then attention can be focused on iatrogenic morbidity and mortality. Figure 21.1 shows that enteric injury is strongly dependent on physique: thin women are a higher risk for small bowel obstruction. This is particularly true for the long-term survivors. All seven UMH complications occurred in cured women. It is possible that patients with more advanced cancers may not live long enough to have a high incidence of chronic radiation injury or may have enteric damage concealed by recurrent tumour. The sample size of the study is too small to draw any further conclusions regarding this issue in view of the prognostic importance of stage, grade, extent of residual tumour, and cell type. If a patient has a very high risk of radiation injury on the basis of thin physique or surgery (Table 21.2), then chemotherapy could be recommended.

Heavy body habitus predisposes to leukaemia when chemotherapy is administered on a milligram per kilogram or a milligram per metre squared basis (Fig. 21.2). The MDAH regimen, for example, prescribed 1 mg per kg for 12 cycles [6]. Thus, a patient weighing 58 or more kilograms would have a 16% leukaemia risk, and a patient weighing 67 or more kilograms would have a 33% leukaemia risk. Doses could be reduced by giving alkylating agents on an ideal weight basis, but if chemotherapy or radiotherapy doses are inordinately lowered, cure rates will probably fall.

Body habitus thus emerges as a possible selection factor between radiation and chemotherapy. The probability estimates of the logistic model and the leukaemia studies are not extremely accurate, but they can be used as a guide. Thin patients could receive chemotherapy, heavy patients could receive radiotherapy, and perhaps intermediate patients could receive both. The chronic toxicities of radiation and Alkeran are additive rather than synergistic: the incidence of neither acute leukaemia nor small bowel obstruction is raised when these agents are administered sequentially [10]. Another alternative is substitution of other chemotherapeutic agents, but these in turn introduce additional risks. Cyclophosphamide, for example, has been associated with the induction of squamous cell carcinomas of the skin and carcinomas of the urinary bladder, as well as acute myeloid leukaemia, with average latent periods of 18 to 81 months [13].

After establishing complication probabilities, the next step is assessment of relevant severity or cost. Any fatal complication has been arbitrarily assigned a value of 100, although it is possible that either leukaemia or bowel injury may cause a death associated with more suffering and thus have a slightly different value. Enteric morbidity is difficult to quantitate but can certainly be substantial. One approach to assigning values could be discussion between the patient and her physician before the initiation of therapy. If this can be done and if the appropriate probabilities can be obtained, then the optimal course of action will be clear.

The limitations of decision theory must not be ignored. The probabilities are only probabilities: they are not certainties. No model can guarantee that the desired outcome will occur. In addition, as shown by the magnitude of the standard deviations of Table 21.3, the predicted probabilities will themselves contain an element of uncertainty. In general, the lower that a predicted complication probability is, the more accurate will be the prediction. Thus, greater faith should be placed in lower rather than higher complication probabilities (Table 21.3).

A second caveat is that some values may be very difficult to quantify. Values are subject to change with the passage of time. It is also very difficult to include all possible values, and the summation of values can be quite complex. The values of the patient and physician are not necessarily the same. Thus, decision theory has two levels of utility. Accurate delineation of complication probabilities for individual patients is intrinsically useful. In addition, if values can be assigned to the costs of relevant outcomes, then decision theory can more clearly show optimal pathways through the maze of cancer management.

Acknowledgement. This work was partly supported by Grant Number CA-15548 from the National Cancer Institute.

References

1. Dembo AJ (1982) The role of radiotherapy in ovarian cancer. Bull Cancer (Paris) 69:275–283
2. Delclos L, Dembo AJ (1980) Female pelvis: ovaries. In: Fletcher GH (ed) Textbook of Radiotherapy, Lea & Febiger, Philadelphia, 3rd edn. pp 834–851
3. Potish RA, Twiggs LB, Adcock LL, Prem KA (to be published) Logistic models for prediction of enteric morbidity in the treatement of ovarian and cervical cancers. J Obstet Gynecol
4. Cox DR (1969) The analysis of binary data. Methuen, London, pp 87–91
5. Greene MH, Boice JD Jr, Greer BE, Blessing JA, Dembo AJ (1982) Acute nonlymphocytic leukemia after therapy with alkylating agents for ovarian cancer: A study of five randomized clinical trials. New Engl J Med 307:1416–1421
6. Smith JP, Rutledge FN, Delclos L (1975) Postoperative treatment of early cancer of the ovary: A random trial between postoperative irradiation and chemotherapy, Natl Cancer Inst Monogr 42:149–153
7. Einhorn N (1978) Acute leukemia after chemotherapy (melphalan). Cancer 41:444–447
8. Chernoff H, Moses LE (1959) Elementary decision theory. Wiley, New York, pp 1–11
9. Smith JP, Rutledge F (1970) Chemotherapy in the treatment of cancer of the ovary, Am J Obstet Gynecol 107:691–703
10. Potish R, Adcock L, Brooker D, Jones TK Jr, Levitt SH, Okagaki T, Prem K (1980) Sequential surgery, radiation therapy, and Alkeran in the management of epithelial carcinoma of the ovary. Cancer 45:2754–2758
11. Brady LW, Blessing JA, Slayton RE, Homesley HD, Lewis GC (1979) Radiotherapy (RT), chemotherapy (CT), and combined therapy in Stage III epithelial ovarian cancer, Cancer Clin Trials 2:111–120
12. Omura GA, Morrow CP, Blessing JA, Miller A, Buchsbaum HJ, Homesley HD, Leone L (1983) A randomized comparison of melphalan versus melphalan plus hexamethylmelamine versus adriamycin plus cyclophosphamide in ovarian cancer. Cancer 51:783–789
13. Schmähl D, Habs M, Lorenz M, Wagner I (1982) Occurrence of second tumors in man after anticancer drug treatment. Cancer Treat Rev 9:167–194

22 · The Use of Pig Lymph Node Cells in the Treatment of Carcinoma of the Ovary

G.M. Turner, V. Barley, E.R. Davies, T. Lai, D. Morris and
M.O. Symes

Introduction

Studies on the use of foreign immunologically competent cells to transfer adoptive immunity to animals and patients with tumours have been in progress since 1960. The initial experiments were carried out using allogeneic (mouse) lymphoid cells [1] or xenogeneic (rat) cells [2] to treat mouse tumours growing in isogeneic hosts. It was found that tumour-immune lymphoid cells were necessary to produce an anti-tumour effect. As a prelude to clinical studies, the pig (which is readily available, cheap, and free from infection) was used as a donor of mesenteric lymph node cells (LNC) in the treatment of mouse tumours growing in isogeneic hosts [3,4]. Mice received mammary carcinoma cells by i.v. injection and 7 days later the resultant experimental pulmonary tumours were treated by i.v. injection of pig LNC. No therapeutic effect was obtained unless the tumour-bearing mice were subject to splenectomy or local thoracic irradiation on day 3 (that is 4 days before the injection of pig LNC), both of which procedures concentrated ^{51}Cr-labelled pig LNC in the lungs. Under these conditions pig LNC immune to the mouse tumour or to mouse skin, but not to a human tumour, produced a significant reduction in the number of pulmonary tumours counted on day 14 (i.e. 7 days after injection of pig LNC). Mouse tumour immune pig LNC injected intraperitoneally (rather than i.v.) so that they did not make immediate contact with the tumours in the mouse lungs were ineffective. When tumour-immune pig LNC were fractionated on a ficolltriosil gradient, fractions containing blast cells were the most effective in producing an anti-tumour effect [5].

At the clinical level each of 77 patients with invasive transitional cell carcinoma

(TCC) of the urinary bladder received a single intra-arterial injection of autoch-
thonous tumour-immune pig LNC into the arterial blood supply of the tumour [6].
The patients were divided into 4 groups, (1) those receiving pig LNC as the only
treatment (16 patients); (2) those who received pig LNC on relapse (judged by
EUA cystoscopy and biopsy) following radical radiotherapy with 5500 cGy (34
patients); (3) those who received pig LNC followed after an interval of 6 weeks by
radiotherapy with 4000 cGy (10 patients); (4) as in group (3) but with the dose of
radiotherapy increased to 5500 cGy (17 patients). Complete remission was
characterised by complete disappearance of the tumour (for a varying time)
following treatment. Partial remission was defined as a reduction in the level of
symptoms and a decrease in tumour size on EUA and/or cystoscopy. There were 1
complete and 3 partial remissions among the patients in group (1), 5 complete and
7 partial in group (2), 6 complete and 2 partial in group (3), 8 complete and 1
partial in group (4). Of the 20 patients showing complete remission, 7 lived for
more than 5 years after treatment.

In a similar study [7] Cockett and his group in Rochester, NY, treated 33
patients with invasive TCC of the bladder by injection of tumour immune pig
lymph node cells. In 8 this was followed by local irradiation and total cystectomy,
and 6 of these patients are alive without evidence of tumour in excess of 1 year
after immunotherapy. A further 4 patients received pig cells in the treatment of
tumour recurrence following radical radiotherapy. Of these, two showed marked
tumour necrosis or complete tumour remission at cystectomy 23 and 32 months
later. Of 10 patients receiving immunotherapy and irradiation only (as cystectomy
was contraindicated by the extent of the tumour), 5 lived in excess of 2 years.
Finally in 11 similar cases receiving immunotherapy alone there were 2 patients
whose expected survival time was prolonged, to 20 and 26 months post-treatment.

Thus the experience in Bristol and Rochester is complementary. Complete
disease remission is seen in some patients with tumour recurrence following
radical radiotherapy, following administration of tumour-immune pig LNC as a
sole treatment.

The present paper describes the treatment of stage III or IV carcinoma of the
ovary, using pig LNC. Carcinoma of the ovary seemed particularly suitable for
this form of immunotherapy as the frequent presence of ascitic fluid containing
free tumour cells would afford a ready means of obtaining pig-cell/tumour-cell
contact following intraperitoneal injection of the pig cells. In addition, ovarian
carcinoma usually presents late and the 5-year survival rate for patients at stage 3
and 4 is 11%, so that new approaches to therapy are needed.

Patients and Methods

Patients

A total of 19 patients are treated. They are divided into two groups. The first 5
(Table 22.1) were considered unsuitable for either cytotoxic chemotherapy or
radiotherapy; for example patient 1 was pregnant and patient 5 was cachectic.
These patients therefore received immune pig LNC as their sole additional

Table 22.1. Patients receiving immune pig LNC as sole treatment

Patient No.	Age (years)	Pre-immunotherapy				Immunotherapy	Outcome post-immunotherapy
		Presentation	Treatment	Histology	Initial clinical course		
1.	27	23/40 pregnant, 1/12 increasing dyspnoea. Right pleural effusion contained cells typical of Ca ovary (Fig. 22.2)	Bilateral salpingo-oophorectomy and hysterectomy	Serous papillary cystadeno-carcinoma L. ovary	–	7d post op. skin-immune pig LNC 1.54×10^9 R. pleural cavity, 1.23×10^9 i.v.	d 5–13 enlarged and tender R. cervical and axillary L. nodes. Regression of pleural effusion over 3 months (Fig. 22.1). Alive and well after 10 years
2.	54	Abdominal swelling and ascites. Lower abdominal mass. Enlarged L. supra-clavicular node	Laparotomy, partial debulking.	Poorly differentiated adenocarcinoma	–	7d post op. tumour immune pig LNC 3.06×10^9 aorta	Remained free of ascites for 2 months. At 4/12 treosulphan. 500 mg bd and DXR to abdomen. Died 6 months progressive disease
3.	69	Abdominal mass	Biopsy—omental mass and peritoneal seedlings	Mod. differentiated adenocarcinoma	–	1 month post-op. skin-immune pig LNC 1.74×10^9 sup. mes. artery, 1.02×10^9 i.p.	At 2 months well, wt. gain 10 lb. At 4 months ascites and intestinal obstruction. Died 6 months progressive disease

Table 22.1. Patients receiving immune pig LNC as sole treatment (*continued*)

Patient No.	Age (years)	Pre-immunotherapy Presentation	Treatment	Histology	Initial clinical course	Immunotherapy	Outcome post-immunotherapy
4.	56	Lower abdominal pain. Swollen L.leg	BSO and TAH, residual metastases in POD and aortic nodes	Papillary carcinoma of ovary	At 4 months sub-acute intestinal obstruction	4 months post-op. skin-immune pig LNC 1.22×10^9 L. int. iliac artery, 1.08×10^9 R. int. iliac artery	At 2 weeks pulmonary embolus, died. Recent haemorrhagic necrosis in pelvic tumour mass.
5.	60	Abdominal swelling, ascites, cachectic	Laparoscopy, biopsy, multiple peritoneal deposits	Serous papillary cystadeno-carcinoma	–	1 month post biopsy skin-immune pig LND 0.75×10^9 R. int. iliac artery, 0.75×10^9 L. int. iliac artery, 0.75×10^9 i.p.	At 6 months well gaining wt. no recurrence of ascites. At 9 months pelvic mass cystic. At 1 yr 6 months enlarging pelvic mass – commenced treosulphan – no response. Died 2 years progressive disease

treatment. The 14 patients in the second group were referred for immunotherapy after they had received all possible chemotherapy and radiotherapy, and at a time when their disease was progressive. They were assigned at random to receive non-immune pig LNC ($n=6$, Table 22.2) or immune pig LNC from animals wherein fragments of the patients' skin or tumour had previously been implanted into the mesentery ($n=8$, Table 22.3).

Immunisation of the Pigs

Approximately 0.5 g of macroscopically viable tumour or four 1 cm^2 pieces of full thickness abdominal skin from the patient were implanted into multiple pockets made between the leaves of the ileal mesentery in a pig. Seven days later the draining mesenteric lymph nodes were harvested.

Preparation of Pig LNC Suspensions

The nodes were chopped into fragments using scissors. These fragments were then reduced to a cell suspension in TCM 199 (with antibiotics) Gibco by gentle grinding in a hand operated glass piston blender. The cell suspension was filtered through 200 stainless steel mesh (to remove embolic cell clumps), washed once (170 g for 5 min) in TCM 199 and suspended in 100 ml TCM 199. The number of total and viable (excluding 0.17% w/v Trypan blue) nucleated cells were counted using a haemocytometer.

Injection of Pig LNC

Immediately prior to injection the LNC were again filtered through 200 gauge mesh. The cells were injected under radiological control via a catheter inserted into the femoral artery and passed retrogradely so that it was positioned in the artery indicated in the tables.

Results and Discussion

Of the five patients in the first group (Table 22.1), two, numbers 1 and 5, showed unequivocal evidence of disease remission. The response in patient 1, who is alive and well after 10 years, should be interpreted with caution, as she was pregnant and apart from her pleural effusion, had stage Ia disease. However, her effusion contained cells that were categorised as malignant by two independent cytologists. Also the association of cervical and axillary lymph node enlargement with disappearance of the effusion, in the 3-month period following pig cell injection, is unlikely to be accidental (see Figs. 22.1, 22.2).

Table 22.2. Patients receiving non-immune pig LNC

Patient No.	Age (years)	Pre-immunotherapy				Immunotherapy	Outcome post-immunotherapy
		Presentation	Treatment	Histology	Initial clinical course	Initial Immunotherapy	
1.	55	Abdominal swelling. At laparotomy unresectable primary tumour with widespread peritoneal dissemination	Chemotherapy. Cisplatinum 20 mg i.v. + treosulphan 500 mg tds, 6 courses over 3 months	Undifferentiated papillary adeno-carcinoma	At 5 months reduction in tumour size. At 6 months tumour growth recommenced. At 8 months pt. cachectic	At 8 months 2.05×10^9 R. int. iliac artery	No recurrence of ascites but no reduction in tumour size. Died 4 months progressive disease
2.	51	Abdominal swelling, dysuria, dyspnoea. Laparotomy—bil. ovarian tumours, metastases in peritoneal cavity, omentum and liver	At 1 month 3700 cGy to pelvis 22 fractions over 42 d. At 1 year cisplatinum 5 courses	Poorly differentiated papillary adenocarcinoma	Reduction in ascites	At 1 year 8 months 0.95×10^9 R. int. iliac 0.95×10^9 L. int. iliac	No response Died 2 months progressive disease
3.	64	Abdominal pain, vaginal bleeding. Laparotomy— multiple intra-peritoneal tumours	Intrauterine radium implant, TAH and BSO	Clear cell carcinoma of mesonephric duct	No response, persistent ascites	At 6 months 0.26×10^9 R. int. iliac, 0.26×10^9 L. int. iliac, 0.26×10^9 i.p.	At 2 months ultrasound— reduction in size of solid tumours. Died 4 months progressive disease

Table 22.2. (*continued*)

| Patient No. | Age (years) | Pre-immunotherapy | | | Initial clinical course | Immunotherapy | Outcome post-immunotherapy |
		Presentation	Treatment	Histology			
4.	60	Wt. loss, abdominal pain, constipation, ascites. Laparotomy—Ca ovary (left), metastases peritoneal cavity, omentum, diaphragm, liver	TAH, BSO. Cisplatinum, chlorambucil 4 courses	Well differentiated papillary cystadeno-carcinoma	No response. At 6 months ascites, pelvic mass	At 6 months 0.73×10^9 R. int. iliac, 0.73×10^9 L. int. iliac, 0.73×10^9 i.p.	No response. At 2 weeks died progressive disease
5.	58	Abdominal pain, constipation. Laparotomy—L. ovarian Ca, metastases in omentum, abdominal wall and liver and on the diaphragm. Ascites	Debulking. Bil. oophorectomy and omentectomy. Cisplatinum 5 courses	Poorly differentiated adenocarcinoma	At 2 months and 5 months sub-acute intestinal obstruction. At 6 months ascites and intra-abdominal tumour masses	At 6 months 0.54×10^9 R. int. iliac, 0.41×10^9 L. int. iliac, 0.41×10^9 i.p.	No response. Died day 9
6.	50	Abdominal mass. Ascites. Laparotomy—Bil. ovarian Ca, metastases in peritoneal cavity, para-aortic lymph nodes, R. kidney and liver	Treosulfan and prednisolone	Granulosa cell Ca of ovary	Well for 9 months then recurrent ascites	At 10 months 1.22×10^9 i.p.	No response. Died at 1 month progressive disease

Table 22.3. Patients given immune pig LNC (implanted skin or tumour)

Patient No.	Age (years)	Pre-immunotherapy Presentation	Treatment	Histology	Initial clinical course	Immunotherapy	Outcome post-immunotherapy
1.	45	Abdominal pain. Vaginal discharge. Laparotomy—bil. ovarian tumours, metastases in peritoneal cavity and omentum	TAH and BSO cisplatinum, vinblastine 4 courses. At 5 months 3000 cGy to abdomen. At 1 year 1 month isofosfamide. At 1 yr 6 months ^{137}Cs insertion p.v.	Poorly differentiated adenocarcinoma	At 1 year 2nd laparotomy metastases in peritoneal cavity At 1 yr 8 months pelvic and vaginal tumours.	At 1 yr 8 months 3.65×10^9 L. int. iliac	Slow deterioration. Died 6 months progressive disease
2.	49	Ca of R. ovary found at cholecystectomy. Metastases in peritoneal cavity and omentum	Cisplatinum 7 courses over 6 months	Poorly differentiated papillary cystadeno-carcinoma	At 7 months dyspnoea, R. pleural effusion, ascites, intra-peritoneal, tumour mass, enlarged R. and L. inguinal nodes	At 8 months, laparotomy 0.49×10^9 tumour mass, 0.49×10^9 L. int. iliac, 0.49×10^9 R. int. iliac, 0.49×10^9 i.p., 0.13×10^9 i.v.	For 1 month necrotic discharge from wound. At 2 months general condition much improved. No ascites, abdominal mass unchanged. At 3 months R. pleural effusion, skin metastases. Died. Autopsy: pelvic tumour completely necrotic

Table 22.3. (*continued*)

| Patient No. | Age (years) | Pre-immunotherapy | | Histology | Initial clinical course | Immunotherapy | Outcome post-immunotherapy |
		Presentation	Treatment				
3.	34	Abdominal pain. Laparotomy—R. ovarian tumour, excised	Cisplatinum 5 courses – 3 months. At 5 months L. oophorectomy, sub-total hysterectomy	Poorly differentiated papillary adenocarcinoma	At 1 month ascites. At 3 months complete remission. At 5 months laparotomy—metastases intraperitoneal, omental, and on L. ovary. At 7 months sub-acute intestinal obstruction	At 8 months 2.7×10^9 R. int. iliac, 2.7×10^9 L. int. iliac	Died 2 months progressive disease
4.	52	Menorrhagia. Ascites. Laparotomy—metastases, intraperitoneal and hepatic	Bil. oophorectomy and debulking of tumour. At 2 months chlorambucil and prednisolone. At 1 yr 9 months 5000 cGy to pelvis. At 1 yr 11 months Treosulphan	Clear cell adenocarcinoma	Remission for 1 year 6 months, disease well controlled. At 1 year 6 months further growth of pelvic tumour. At 2 year 6 months complete remission. At 2 year 9 months recurrent pelvic tumour. At 3 year 2 months multiple hepatic metastases	At 3 yr 3 months 2.85×10^9 R. hepatic, 1.27×10^9 R. int. iliac, 1.27×10^9 L. int. iliac	On day 16 gastro-enterostomy for pyloric stenosis. Multiple viable hepatic metastases. Died 3 yr 5 months progressive disease

Table 22.3. (*continued*)

Patient No.	Age (years)	Pre-immunotherapy		Histology	Initial clinical course	Immunotherapy	Outcome post-immunotherapy
		Presentation	Treatment				
5.	58	Abdominal pain. Ascites. Laparotomy—multiple intraperitoneal tumours, ovarian primary	Treosulphan	Poorly differentiated papillary adenocarcinoma	Remission for 9 months. At 10 months, ascites, multiple intra-peritoneal tumour masses	At 10 months 1.5 × 10⁹ R. int. iliac, 1.5 × 10⁹ L. int. iliac, 2.45 × 10⁹ i.p.	At 1 month ascites, pleural effusion, thiotepa. Died 2 months progressive disease
6.	63	Ascites. Abdominal mass. Laparotomy—fixed Ca L. ovary, metastases in omentum, peritoneal cavity and liver	Treosulphan 8 courses – 1 yr 8 months	Poorly differentiated adenocarcinoma	Remission for 1 yr 8 months. At 2nd laparotomy ascites metastases in peritoneal cavity, omentum and liver	At 1 yr 9 months 0.74 × 10⁹ Sub. mes. artery, 1.23 × 10⁹ L. int. iliac	No response. Died 3 months
7.	43	Wt. loss. Ascites Laparotomy—Ca of both ovaries, metastases in omentum	TAH and BSO Cisplatinum and treosulphan 4 courses in 2 months. 4750 cGy to abdomen 20 fractions. At 1 year Treosulphan	Papillary adenocarcinoma	At 9 months ileo-ilial anastamosis for intestinal obstruction due to recurrent pelvic tumour with multiple metastases. At 1 yr 7 months 3rd laparotomy for intestinal obstruction, no bypass possible	At 1 yr 8 months 1.52 × 10⁹ R. int. iliac, 1.52 × 10⁹ L. int. iliac	No response. Died 1 month
8.	54	Abdominal pain, ascites, palpable pelvic and abdominal tumours	–	From ascitic fluid, adenocarcinoma cells	–	At 1 month 1.5 × 10⁹ L. int. iliac, 0.8 × 10⁹ R. int. iliac, 1.13 × 10⁹ i.p.	No response. At 2 weeks died

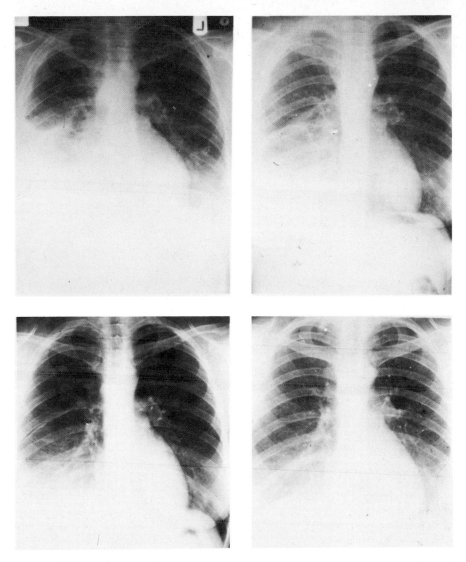

Fig. 22.1. Patient 1 (Table 22.1). Serial chest radiography taken before immunotherapy (*top left*) and at intervals of 3 weeks (*top right*); 7 weeks (*bottom left*) and 14 weeks (*bottom right*). There is progressive resolution of the right pleural effusion.

In patients 2 and 3 (group 1), progress of the disease was slowed, as judged by the delay (2/12) in re-accumulation of previous ascites.

The patients in group 2 were entered into a controlled trial to compare the effect of non-immune with immune pig LNC. As may be seen from Tables 22.2 and 22.3 all of these patients had advanced disease and some were in a terminal condition. None of these patients showed evidence of disease remission.

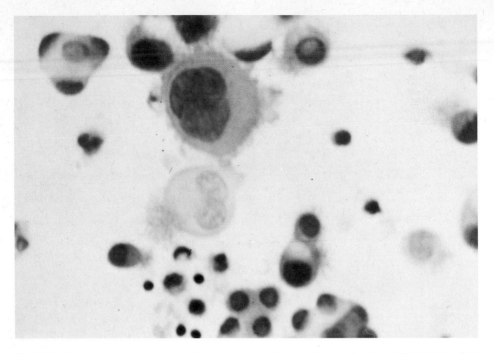

Fig. 22.2. A cytospin preparation of cells from the right pleural effusion of patient 1 (Table 22.1). Cells typical of a serous papillary cystadenocarcinoma of the ovary, with 'brush' borders, are seen. (H & E, × 500.)

There was a marked contrast in the outcome of treating patients de novo or following chemo/radiotherapy, with pig LNC. In part this may reflect the more advanced disease in the second group of patients.

In vitro studies [8] did not demonstrate any cytotoxicity of either non-immune or immune pig LNC for human peripheral blood lymphocytes or tumour cells. Thus any antitumour action of the pig LNC may depend on the involvement of the tumour as a 'bystander' in the rejection by the patient of tumour infiltrating pig cells. Thus, to facilitate localisation of pig LNC in the tumour, the cells were administered via its arterial blood supply, or into a malignant cell containing effusion.

The patients in group 2 had received previous immunosuppressive chemo/radiotherapy. Thus they may have responded less to the presence of pig cells so that no antitumour effect was observed.

It would be desirable to compare the efficacy of immunotherapy when given before or after chemo/radiotherapy in a prospective controlled trial.

Acknowledgements. This work was supported by the Cancer Research Campaign and the Bristol and Weston Health Authority.

References

1. Woodruff MFA, Symes MO (1962) The use of immunologically competent cells in the treatment of cancer: Experiments with a transplantable mouse tumour. Br J Cancer 16:707–715
2. Woodruff MFA, Symes MO, Stuart AE (1963) The effect of rat spleen cells on two transplanted mouse tumours. Br J Cancer 17:320–327
3. Prichard-Thomas S, Symes MO (1978) The use of immunologically competent cells from pig mesenteric lymph nodes to treat pulmonary tumours in mice. Cancer Immunol Immunother 5:129–133
4. Prichard-Thomas S, Symes MO (1978) Observations on the effect of radiotherapy followed by injection of pig lymph node cells, in reducing the number of pulmonary tumours induced by intravenous injection of tumour cells into isogenic mice. Cancer Immunol Immunother 5:135–139
5. Khezri AA, Lai T, Symes MO (1984) The use of pig mononuclear cells to inhibit pulmonary tumour formation in isogeneic mice. J Surg Res 37:354–360
6. Symes MO, Eckert H, Feneley RCL et al. (to be published) The treatment of bladder carcinoma with tumour-immune pig lymph node cells—a Phase 1 study. Urology
7. Cockett ATK, Di Sant' Agnese PA, Hamlin DJ, Keys HM (1982) Porcine sensitized lymph node cells (immunotherapy) and attenuated irradiation for infiltrative transitional cell carcinoma of bladder. Urology 19:593–598
8. Morris DM, Heinemann D, Symes MO (1984) The in vitro reactivity of pig lymph node cells (LNC) against human target cells. J Exp Clin Cancer Res 3:39–47

23 · Carcinoma of the Ovary and Serum Lactic Dehydrogenase Levels with Emphasis on Dysgerminoma

G.M. Awais

Patient Study

I have reported that serum lactic dehydrogenase (SLDH) appears to be elevated in the presence of primary carcinoma of the ovary, but not in other pelvic tumours, benign or malignant [1]. A retrospective study was done of 43 primary carcinomas of the ovary treated at the Cleveland Clinic for about 3–4 years. Of the 43 patients, 23 had some form of treatment before coming to the Clinic, and 20 were treated at the Clinic. Of these 20, 6 had SLDH determinations both before and after treatment, 8 after treatment only, and 6 before treatment only.

The histopathological findings in these 20 patients were as follows:

Pathology	No of patients
Papillary adenocarcinoma	12
9 poorly differentiated	
2 moderately differentiated	
1 well differentiated	
Papillary mucinous cystadenocarcinoma	4
Papillary serous cystadenocarcinoma	4

The FIGO (International Federation of Gynecology and Obstetrics) ovarian cancer staging of these 20 cases were as follows: stage I, 3 patients; stage III, 15 patients; stage IV, 2 patients.

Results

The six patients in whom SLDH was determined before and after treatment showed that SLDH levels were higher than normal before treatment. After treatment, the SLDH levels decreased to values within or close to normal limits. In eight patients, the SLDH was determined after treatment only, and the SLDH levels were all within normal range. In the remaining six patients, SLDH levels were determined before treatment only and the levels were higher than normal.

A prospective study was then done on 18 patients [2]. Each patient was found to have a pelvic mass in which neoplasm was suspected. Ten were found to have different stages of carcinoma of the ovary and had elevated SLDH levels pre-operatively (Table 23.1). Postoperatively, SLDH levels showed a sharp reduction in all but two patients. Patient 7 had the operation at another hospital and no postoperative SLDH was done. Patient 8 underwent laparotomy only and the extent of the disease precluded further operation.

The remaining eight patients had benign diseases (Table 23.2); none had carcinoma of the ovary. Despite the varied pathology in the uterus or adnexae, SLDH levels were not elevated in the absence of carcinoma of the ovary.

In a recent study at the Cleveland Clinic of 22 patients with seminoma of the testis, mediastinal germinoma, and ovarian dysgerminoma, we determined the levels of SLDH both before and after treatment [3]. Six women had ovarian dysgerminoma, four men had mediastinal seminoma and the remaining 12 patients had testicular seminoma. The 12 men with testicular seminoma came to the clinic for follow-up care only, after having undergone treatment elsewhere. No SLDH determinations were therefore available for these patients and they were not considered in the study. In the four patients with mediastinal germinoma, the SLDH levels were elevated before treatment and dropped towards normal levels after treatment (Table 23.3).

In the six patients with ovarian dysgerminoma, the SLDH levels before treatment were highly elevated and reduced to within normal after treatment (Table 23.4).

Table 23.1. Carcinoma of the ovary and histopathological findings

Patient No.	Age (yrs)	Stage	Histopathological findings
1	53	IIb	Papillary adenocarcinoma, poorly differentiated
2	51	III	Papillary serous cystadenocarcinoma
3	45	IV	Papillary adenocarcinoma
4	54	III	Poorly differentiated adenocarcinoma
5	56	III	Poorly to partially differentiated papillary cystadenocarcinoma
6	58	IIIa	Papillary serous cystadenocarcinoma
7	55	IIIb	Adenocarcinoma
8	67	IV	Adenocarcinoma
9	60	IV	Adenocarcinoma of ovary, involving colon
10	17	Ic	Dysgerminoma of right ovary. Uterus, tubes and left ovary showed no significant change. Omentum negative for carcinoma; pelvic and para-aortic lymph nodes negative for carcinoma. Pelvic washings showed malignant cells

Table 23.2. Pathological conditions of organs of the pelvis, other than carcinoma of the ovary

Patient No	Age (yrs)	Histopathological findings
11	71	Adenocarcinoma endometrium, diffuse haemorrhage of left ovary. Adenofibroma of right ovary
12	24	Cystic teratoma, left ovary
13	59	Fibroma of right ovary
14	70	Benign sex mesenchymoma growing principally as a Sertoli cell tumour
15	45	Serous cystadenoma, left ovary. Tubo-ovarian abscess. Chronic cystic salpingitis
16	54	Malignant mixed tumour of the mesoderm, right adnexa. No carcinoma, or involvement, of the ovary
17	71	Diverticulitis with colovesical fistula
18	72	Giant multilocular mucinous cystadenoma, right ovary, 13 by 14 cm, weight 13.6 kg; leiomyoma, subserosal

Table 23.3. Mediastinal germinomas, male patients

Patient No.	Age (yrs)	Histopathological findings	SLDH (mU/ml) Before treatment	After treatment
1	22	Malignant neoplasm strongly suggestive of seminoma of mediastinum	300	100
2	44	Anaplastic seminoma of mediastinum	380	NA
3	52	Mixed germinoma, seminoma and choriocarcinoma of mediastinum	>500	150
4	30	Mediastinal seminoma	900	150

Table 23.4. Dysgerminoma of the ovary

Patient No.	Age (yrs)	Histopathological findings	Stage	SLDH (mU/ml) Before treatment	After treatment
1	20	Dysgerminoma of left ovary	I	280	Normal
2	21	Dysgerminoma of right ovary	I	2335	Normal
3	17	Dysgerminoma of right ovary	Ic	1950	Normal
4	18	Dysgerminoma of left ovary	IIb	NA	Normal
5	25	Dysgerminoma of left ovary	Ia	603	Normal
6	28	Dysgerminoma of left ovary	Ia	1260	Normal

Discussion

In normal tissue, the glycolytic activity is much less than in malignant tissue. About 60 years ago, Warburg and Minami [4] and Cori and Cori [5] demonstrated that malignant tissue has high glycolytic activity.

The anaerobic conversion of glucose to lactic acid is called glycolysis, and pyruvate is the end product of this carbohydrate metabolism. Pyruvate is catalysed by the major enzyme lactic dehydrogenase to form lactate, which is a reversible reaction. With increased glycolytic activity, which occurs in malignant tissue, one would expect a concomitant increase in LDH enzyme activity. The increase in LDH level may be reflected in tissue fluids and may then be measured.

The ovary, a multipotential organ may, during malignant proliferation, show exceptionally increased LDH activity, which can then be measured in the circulating plasma. Results of studies seem to confirm this hypothesis.

SLDH had been reported to be elevated in patients with lymphoma, granulocytic leukaemia, carcinoma of the pancreas and gall bladder, metastasis from carcinoma of the breast, and metastatic disease of the liver. It is also elevated in cases of myocardial infarction, infectious mononucleosis, thrombocytopenia, obstructive jaundice, and acute hepatitis [6–9].

Based on the findings in our studies, it appears that the enzyme SLDH is elevated in the presence of carcinoma of the ovary, particularly dysgerminoma of the ovary. Further studies are needed to clarify the relationship of SLDH and carcinoma of the ovary.

References

1. Awais GM (1973) Serum lactic dehydrogenase levels in the diagnosis and treatment of carcinoma of the ovary. Am J Obstet Gynecol 116:1053–1057
2. Awais GM (1978) Carcinoma of the ovary and serum lactic dehydrogenase levels. Surg Gynecol Obstet 146:893–895
3. Awais GM (1983) Dysgerminoma and serum lactic dehydrogenase levels. Obstet Gynecol 61:99–101
4. Warburg O, Minami S (1923) Experiments on surviving carcinomatous tissue. Klin Wochenschr 2:776–777
5. Cori CF, Cori GT (1925) Carbohydrate metabolism of tumors; changes in sugar, lactic acid, and CO_2-combining power of blood passing through tumor. J Biol Chem 65:398–405
6. Hsieh KM, Blumenthal HT (1956) Serum lactic dehydrogenase levels in various disease states. Proc Soc Exp Biol Med 91:626–630
7. Wroblewski F, LaDue JS (1955) Lactic dehydrogenase activity in blood. Proc Soc Exp Biol Med 90:210–213
8. Wroblewski F, Gregory KF (1961) Lactic dehydrogenase isoenzymes and their distribution in normal tissues and plasma and in disease states. Ann NY Acad Sci 94:912–932
9. Wroblewski F (1961) Lactic dehydrogenase activity in cancer diagnosis. Med Clin North Am 45:513–520

24 · Combination Chemotherapy of Ovarian Carcinoma with Cisplatinum and Treosulphan — A Phase II Study*

I.D. Duncan and L.A. Clayton

Introduction

Ovarian carcinoma continues to be a major problem as well as a challenge for the medical staff involved in the care of such patients. It is the most common cause of death from gynaecological malignancy and is the fourth most common cause of death from cancer among British women. Because of the insidious growth of ovarian tumours, a high percentage of patients will have advanced disease at the time of diagnosis. Until recently, survivals were disappointing with 5 years survival in stage I being 50%–65%, stage II 38%–60% and stage III 5%–10% [1]. Historically, the alkylating agents have been the mainstay of postoperative treatment for ovarian carcinoma. However, complete response rates with single agent therapy have been low. Regimens employing cisplatinum and its analogues have recently been associated with an increased response rate and thereby an opportunity for increased survival [2]. Treosulphan, a bifunctional alkylating agent was introduced in the United Kingdom in 1976 following 10 years' use in Scandinavia. It has been shown to achieve high response rates as a single agent, to be well tolerated by the patient, to induce minimal nausea, no alopecia and has excellent effects on ascites and pleural effusions, its main side effect being myelotoxicity [3–6]. Sensitivity studies in animal tumour lines have shown that combinations of cisplatinum and treosulphan produce longer remissions than either agent alone, with no evidence of increased toxicity [7].

* To be published in the *British Journal of Obstetrics and Gynaecology* and included by kind permission of the editors.

At the beginning of this study, all available data suggested that these drugs were active against epithelial ovarian carcinoma as single agents. It was therefore hypothesised that they should make a good combination drug regimen. Our aims were to: (a) induce a remission with the cisplatinum and treosulphan combination; (b) consolidate the remission with treosulphan alone; (c) re-appraise the situation at the end of one year to evaluate the need for further chemotherapy; and (d) minimise side effects.

Patients and Methods

Between April 1981 and December 1983 a total of 60 patients with primary epithelial ovarian carcinoma were diagnosed ante-mortem at Ninewells Hospital and Medical School, Dundee. There were 31 patients with macroscopic disease postoperatively. Eight of these patients were not recruited (2 refused treatment, alternative treatment was chosen for 4, and 2 were considered too debilitated to undergo therapy). A total of 23 patients were therefore recruited, but 2 patients with previous malignancy (one colon, one breast) were excluded from evaluation in this study. There were 17 patients with FIGO stage III disease and one patient with stage IV. There were two patients with stage II disease and one patient with a recurrence. The stage was determined by review of case notes and operative reports. Ideally, FIGO staging implies that a thorough examination of the pelvis and abdominal cavity, retroperitoneal structures, liver and diaphragm is performed. The primary operator was a gynaecologist in 13 cases, a general surgeon assisted by a gynaecologist in three cases and a general surgeon alone in five cases. All surgeons were encouraged to document spread of disease as precisely as possible. Major cytoreductive surgery was deemed possible in only three patients.

On entry into the study all patients underwent clinical examination, chest X-ray, full blood count, blood urea and creatinine, liver function tests and serum electrolytes. With the exception of the chest X-ray, these tests were repeated 4 weeks after each course of chemotherapy and more frequently thereafter if abnormality was detected. The patient characteristics are shown in Table 24.1. No patient was excluded on the basis of age alone.

Postoperatively, the chemotherapy was planned in two phases: the first to consist of six courses of cisplatinum and treosulphan in combination given at monthly intervals, and the second to consist of six courses of treosulphan given as a single agent at monthly intervals. In the first phase, the planned dose schedule was cisplatinum 60 mg/m^2 i.v. on day 1, followed by treosulphan 500 mg twice daily orally on days 3 through 9, the cycle to be repeated every 28 days. Hydration and diuresis were established in all patients by giving 1.5 litres of dextrose in saline i.v. over 9 h. The cisplatinum was administered in divided doses in 2 litres of dextrose in saline over the next 8 h. A diuresis was maintained following therapy with at least 1 litre of dextrose in saline. To minimise nausea and vomiting during and after treatment, one tablet of Motipress was given at night on a continuous basis. Additionally, a variety of anti-emetic agents were employed contemporary with the cisplatinum infusion. Metoclopramide in high doses has recently been the anti-emetic of choice. The plan for the second phase of chemotherapy was

Table 24.1. Clinical characteristics

	Total number
Evaluable patients	21
Age at diagnosis (years)	
Median	60
Range	48–80
FIGO stage	
II	2
III	17
IV	1
Recurrence	1
Histology of tumour	
Mucinous	0
Serous	9
Endometrioid	8
Clear cell	2
Unclassified	2
Grade of tumour	
Moderate	6
Poor	15
Type of operation	
Biopsy only	11
> Biopsy only < TAH, BSO omentectomy	7
TAH, BSO omentectomy	3
Residual disease	
≤2 cm	5
>2 cm	16

treosulphan administered orally as a single agent at doses of 500 mg twice daily on 21 consecutive days out of 28 for a total of six courses.

Follow-up assessment for response included physical examination and ab-domino-pelvic ultrasound. Response criteria were based on the W.H.O. Handbook [8]. A 'complete response' was determined by complete disappearance of all known disease for at least 4 weeks. A 'partial response' was determined if there was an estimated decrease in tumour size by 50% or more for at least 4 weeks. 'No change' implied no significant change for at least 4 weeks. This included 'stable disease', estimated decrease of disease by less than 50% and lesions with an estimated increase of less than 25%. 'Progressive disease' was determined by the appearance of any new lesion not previously identified or an estimated increase of 25% or more in the extent of the lesion. To be included in the study, all patients had to receive at least two courses of therapy. Survival was calculated from the date of initial therapy until death or 30 November 1984. No patients have been lost to follow-up.

All patients who showed a complete clinical response after completing chemotherapy and all patients who had significant partial response after incomplete initial operation, were offered a second-look procedure. Total abdominal hysterectomy, bilateral salpingo-oophorectomy and omentectomy were performed when possible if they had not been performed initially. If laparoscopy was the second-look procedure, then washings were routinely obtained. Actuarial survival curves were calculated for the total group of patients.

Results

The response to treatment is summarised in Table 24.2. The overall response rate by clinical and ultrasound evaluation was 86%, but ultrasound was less optimistic in assessing 'completeness' of response. Clinically, the complete response rate was 14 out of 21 (67%) compared with 10 out of 21 (48%) by ultrasound.

Myelosuppression was the most significant toxicity (Table 24.3), especially during the second phase of chemotherapy when treosulphan was used alone. Six of 21 patients had grade 3/4 myelosuppression in the first phase of chemotherapy with the cisplatinum–treosulphan combination. A delay between courses was necessary in 9 of the 21 patients and in 3 of them the first phase was abandoned because of myelosuppression. One patient continued the first phase on a reduced dose. Sixteen patients received two or more courses of treosulphan alone. Grade 3/4 myelosuppression developed in seven, of whom one had had a similar first phase myelosuppression also. Delay between courses in the second phase was necessary in 12 of the 16 patients. Ten of the 16 had their treosulphan dosage halved and none of the six who had treosulphan in full dosage had more than four courses. As a result of significant leucopenia, two patients developed systemic infections. Both cases were successfully treated with antibiotics. Most patients experienced nausea and vomiting during or immediately after the cisplatinum administration, but only three patients experienced significant nausea and vomiting between courses of treatment. No patient developed alopecia, but two patients had slight hair loss while receiving therapy. The blood urea was mildly elevated in seven patients and the creatinine in two. These patients were judged to have renal toxicity and the treatment was, therefore, aborted. The renal status in these two patients subsequently returned to normal after discontinuing therapy. There were no cases of neurotoxicity or peripheral neuropathy associated with the cisplatinum therapy. Ototoxicity was not subjectively noted in any patient. Routine audiograms were not performed. Of the patients evaluated for the cisplatinum and treosulphan combined regime, 17 completed their therapy while

Table 24.2. Response to therapy
1st phase — cisplatinum and treosulphan in combination

	CR	PR	NC	PD	Total
Clinical	14	4	2	1	21
Ultrasound	10	8	2	1	21

2nd phase — treosulphan as single agent

Ultrasound CR maintained	8
Ultrasound PR maintained	5
Ultrasound CR induced	1
Progressive disease	6
Not given	1
	21

CR = complete response
PR = partial response
NC = no change
PD = progressive disease

Table 24.3. Myelotoxicity

Grade (WHO 1979)	0	1	2	3	4
Haemoglobin (g/100 ml)	≥11	9.5–10.9	8.0–9.4	6.5–7.9	<6.5
1st phase ($n = 21$)[a]	4	5	8	3	1
2nd phase ($n = 16$)[b]	2	6	5	2	1
Leucocytes (1000/mm³)	≥4	3.0–3.9	2.0–2.9	1.0–1.9	<1.0
1st phase	3	5	9	3	1
2nd phase	1	7	2	5	1
Platelets (1000/mm³)	≥100	75–99	50–74	25–49	<25
1st phase	11	3	5	1	1
2nd phase	3	3	4	6	0

[a]   1st phase: cisplatinum and treosulphan in combination
[b]   2nd phase: treosulphan as single agent (for at least two courses)

four cases were aborted (one secondary to renal toxicity, one secondary to both renal toxicity and bone marrow toxicity, and two secondary to bone marrow toxicity with progressive disease). The treosulphan-alone regime was completed in five patients, aborted after two or more courses in 11 (six for second-look laparotomy and five for progressive disease), aborted after a single course in four patients with progressive disease and not prescribed at all to one patient whose disease was also progressing. Blood transfusions were administered to 12 patients.

The performance status was not evaluated objectively in a prospective manner, but subjectively those patients who responded to therapy generally enjoyed a normal lifestyle between courses.

Eleven patients underwent a second-look operation following chemotherapy. Nine of the 11 patients had no clinical evidence of disease prior to their second-look procedure, seven of which were negative and two positive. The details of the surgical procedures and the subsequent outcome are seen in Table 24.4. Nine patients with progressive disease did not undergo further surgery and neither did an octogenarian in complete remission.

The actuarial survival curves are shown in Figs. 24.1–24.3. The overall actuarial survival of all patients evaluated was 24.2% at 43 months (Fig. 24.1) with a median survival of 21 months. There was a 54.9% probability of survival at 43 months in those patients with a complete response, but no patient with a partial response survived beyond 29 months (Fig. 24.2). The complete and partial responders were analysed using the conventional Mantel–Haenszel log-rank test. The survival curves are significantly different ($0.05 > P > 0.01$). One patient's disease progressed while she received the combination chemotherapy and she died at 6 months, and 2 further patients who failed to respond died at 8 and 11 months after an initial period of stable disease. Figure 24.3 shows the survival curves according to the size of the largest portion of residual disease left after the initial operation. These were analysed using a Wilcoxon test which should be more sensitive for early differences, but this failed to reveal any significant difference between the two curves ($P \simeq 0.25$), possibly because of the small numbers involved.

Table 24.4. Surgical reappraisal

Status pre-chemotherapy	Status pre-second-look	Procedure	Findings	Subsequent status
< 2 cm	CR	TAH LSO	Neg.	Recurred 8 months later Died with disease at 17 months
< 2 cm	CR	Laparoscopy Cytology	Neg.	Alive — ? NED 27 months later
< 2 cm	Clinical CR Ultrasound PR	Omentectomy	Neg.	Recurred 9 months later Died Ca. at 10 months
2 cm	CR	Laparotomy Biopsy	Pos.	Died with disease 6 months later
2 cm	CR	Laparoscopy Cytology	Neg.	Alive — NED 31 months later
> 2 cm	CR	TAH	Neg.	Alive — NED 21 months later
> 2 cm	CR	Laparoscopy	Neg.	Recurred 23 months later Alive with disease at 31 months
> 2 cm	CR	TAH	Neg.	Alive — NED 14 months later
> 2 cm	Clinical CR Ultrasound PR	TAH Sigmoid colectomy	Pos.	Died with disease 18 months later
> 2 cm	PR	TAH LSO Omentectomy	Pos.	Died with disease 11 months later
> 2 cm	PD	Palliative	Pos.	Died 48 hours later

CR = Complete response   NED = No evidence of disease
PR = Partial response   TAH = Total abdominal hysterectomy
PD = Progressive disease   LSO = Left salpingo-oophorectomy

Discussion

Significant antitumour activity of cisplatinum against ovarian carcinoma was reported by Wiltshaw and Kroner in 1976 [9]. Since then, it has been used by many investigators in combination with other cytotoxic drugs. A recent review by Neijt [2] indicated that the cumulative response rate with combination chemotherapy not employing cisplatinum was 47% with a median survival of 14 months, while the cumulative response rate of regimens including cisplatinum was 68% with a median survival of 19 months. There have been other reports that indicate response rates with cisplatinum combinations as high as 81% with complete responses of 39% [10,11]. Response rates are improved employing these various combinations, but toxicity continues to be of concern. The ideal drugs used in combination should be those producing effective results as single agents alone without overlapping toxicity. The combination chosen for this study was attractive because cisplatinum and treosulphan appeared to have independent activity as single agents [12], different pharmacological properties and mechanisms of action [13,14] and different patterns of organ toxicity with the exception of myelosuppression [15,16]. Our study objectives, as previously outlined, were achieved to a large degree. A clinical response (complete or partial) was noted in

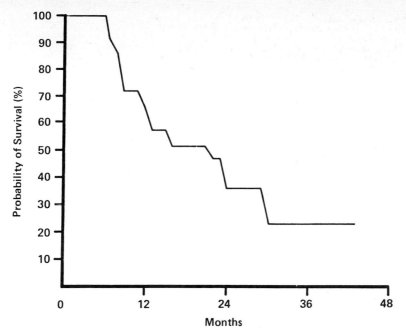

Fig. 24.1. Overall survival; $n = 21 \rightarrow 2$ (15 cancer deaths).

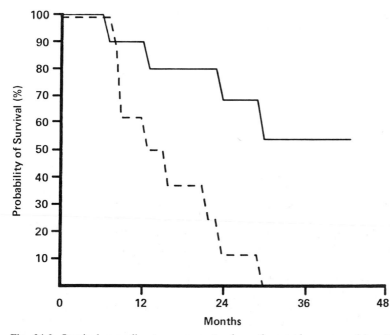

Fig. 24.2. Survival according to response to chemotherapy (as measured by ultrasound). ———— Complete response, $n = 10 \rightarrow 2$ (4 cancer deaths). ————— Partial response, $n = 8 \rightarrow 0$ (8 cancer deaths). $0.05 > P > 0.01$.

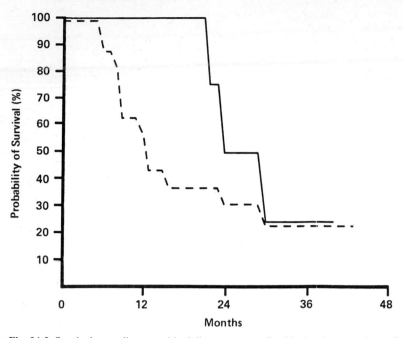

Fig. 24.3. Survival according to residual disease. ———— Residual < 2 cm $n = 5 \rightarrow 1$ (3 cancer deaths).
———— Residual $\geq$ 2 cm $n = 15 \rightarrow 2$ (12 cancer deaths). $P \simeq 0.25$.

18 of 21 patients (86%). The treosulphan maintained a response as judged by ultrasound in 13 of 18 patients (72%) and induced a complete response in one additional patient. Clinically, a complete response was observed in 14 of 21 patients (67%), but complete responses as judged by ultrasound were noted in only 10 of 21 patients (48%). This compares favourably with other reported studies. Subsequent events showed that ultrasound was more accurate in predicting degree of response, but even laparoscopy and laparotomy did not reveal all the disease persisting after chemotherapy.

The only noted toxicity was haematological, especially in the second phase when the treosulphan was used as a single agent. The planned dosage was found to be too high and for most patients 500 mg at night for 21 out of 28 days was more appropriate. With the exception of tiredness induced by anaemia, moderate myelosuppression is largely asymptomatic and so most patients tolerated their chemotherapy well and there were no drug-related deaths.

Recently, Abdullah et al. [17] have achieved the extremely high single agent response rate of 79% using treosulphan intravenously and are now combining it with cisplatinum. Fennelly et al. [18] have also used cisplatinum and treosulphan in combination giving cisplatinum 60 mg i.v. on day one and oral treosulphan 250 mg four times a day for 14 days every 4 weeks. They achieved a response in 17 of 22 patients (77%) with residual disease. We would agree that treosulphan and cisplatinum are a useful combination in the treatment of advanced ovarian cancer. Our data suggest that while short term survival may depend upon the extent of residual disease, longer term survival is determined by response to chemotherapy.

References

1. Tobias JS, Griffiths CT (1976) Management of ovarian carcinoma. N Engl J Med 294:818–822
2. Neijt JP (1983) Combination chemotherapy in the treatment of advanced ovarian carcinoma. I.C.G. Printing, Dordrecht, Netherlands, pp 10–14
3. Fennelly J (1977) Treosulfan (dihydroxybusulphan) in the management of ovarian carcinoma. Br J Obstet Gynaecol 84:300–303
4. Larsen MS (1973) Treosulphan in the treatment of ovarian carcinoma. Acta Obstet Gynecol Scand (suppl.) 22:12–17
5. Lundvall F (1973) Treosulfan in the treatment of ovarian carcinoma. Acta Obstet Gynaecol Scand (suppl.) 22:3–11
6. White WF (1982) Continuous versus intermittent treatment with treosulfan in advanced ovarian cancer. In: Pertiti P, Grassi GG (eds) Current chemotherapy and immunotherapy. Proc. 12 Int. Congress of chemotherapy, Florence, Italy, 9–14 July 1981. Am Soc Mocrobiol pp 1335–1337
7. Preece AW, Wells-Wilson M (1982) Enhancement of responses of a lymphoblastic tumour by combination of the cycle specific drugs cisplatinum and treosulfan. Br J Cancer 46:498
8. WHO (1979) Handbook for reporting results of cancer treatment W.H.O. Offset Publication No. 48
9. Wiltshaw E, Kroner T (1976) Phase II study of cisdichlorodiammineplatinin (II) (NSC – 119873) in advanced adenocarcinoma of the ovary. Cancer Treat Rep 60:55–60
10. Barker GH, Wiltshaw E (1981) Randomised trial comparing low dose cisplatinin and chlorambucil with low dose cisplatinin, chlorambucil and adriamycin in advanced ovarian carcinoma. Lancet I:747–750
11. Ehrlich CE, Einhorn L, Stehman FB, Blessing J (1983) Treatment of advanced epithelial ovarian carcinoma using cisplatinum, adriamycin and cytoxan—The Indiana University experience. Clin Obstet Gynecol 10:325–335
12. Wilson AP, Neal FE (1981) In vitro sensitivity of human ovarian tumours to chemotherapeutic agents. Br J Cancer 44:189–200
13. Drobnik J (1983) Antitumour activity of platinum complexes. Cancer Chemother Pharmacol 10:145–149
14. Feit BW, Rastrup-Anderson N, Matagne R (1970) Studies on epoxide formation from (2S, 3S)-threitol 1, 4-bismethanesulfonate. The preparation and biological activity of (2S, 3S)- 1,2 epoxy 3,4-butanediol 4-methanesulfonate. J Med Chem 13:1173–1175
15. Nadias NE, Harrington JT (1978) Platinum nephrotoxicity. Am J Med 65:307–314
16. White WF (1978) Investigations of response to and complications of treosulfan in the treatment of ovarian tumours. Current Chemother 2:1311–1312
17. Abdullah U, Makanje HH, Cox C, Alsaidi TK, White WF, Masding JE (1983) Chemotherapy of advanced ovarian carcinoma. Use of intravenous treosulfan in previously untreated disease. In: Proceedings of 13th International Congress of Chemotherapy, Vienna, Austria, August 1983
18. Fennelly JJ, Jones B, Cantwell B, Meagher D (1983) Role of second look procedures in evaluating combined treosulfan and cisplatinum in ovarian carcinoma. In: Proceedings of the 13th International Congress of Chemotherapy, Vienna, Austria, August 1983

SECTION V

Vulva

25 · Conservative Management of Vulvar Carcinoma

P. Kolstad, T. Iversen

Introduction

Carcinoma of the vulva constitutes 0.9% of all female malignancies in Norway, and 4.0% of all gynaecological malignancies. Survival studies performed by the Cancer Registry of Norway [1] have shown a significant improvement in prognosis from the years prior to 1962 to the years after 1968 (Fig. 25.1). Since the majority of the patients during this period were treated in the Norwegian Radium Hospital, this improvement in prognosis most probably reflects the fact that from the early 1960s radical vulvectomy with bilateral lymphadenectomy was introduced as standard treatment for all stages. Before this time, treatment was less radical and varied from case to case. Lymphadenectomy was not always performed, and sometimes the patients were given radiotherapy only.

We have reviewed a series of 424 patients with epidermoid carcinoma of the vulva followed for 3–21 years [2]. Using the actuarial life-table technique, the total 5-year survival rate was 67%, 93% in stage I, 75% in stage II, 50% in stage III and 13% in stage IV. The prognosis for the 258 of these patients who were treated with radical vulvectomy and bilateral lymphadenectomy was significantly better. The 5-year survival rate for these patients was 85% in stage II and 65% in stage III.

With these results in mind, the question arises of whether it is advisable to change our treatment policy, a policy which has been followed by a large number of institutions all over the world for about 30 years. However, in the past decade, the terms microinvasive, superficial, and early invasive carcinoma of the vulva have come into use. Wharton, Gallager and Rutledge [3] defined microinvasive vulvar carcinoma as a lesion of diameter less than 2 cm with invasion less than

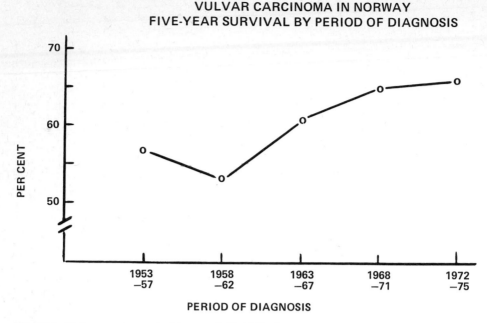

Fig. 25.1. Vulvar carcinoma in Norway, 1953–1975; 5-year survival figures (%) related to each diagnostic period.

5 mm into the stroma. They claimed that such lesions may be treated more conservatively than larger lesions without jeopardising the results.

There is no doubt that standard treatment with radical vulvectomy and bilateral lymphadenectomy is a mutilating procedure, especially in the younger age groups. The immediate postoperative course is frequently complicated by sloughing of the skin, necrosis and infection. Debilitating lymphoedema has been reported in 5%–10%. Sexual activity may be a major problem, especially in the younger age groups. The operation includes extirpation of the Bartholin's gland and the clitoris, and often leads to narrowing of the vaginal introitus. If, therefore, some safe guidelines for a more individualised and conservative approach could be defined, much suffering might be avoided.

Stage I Carcinoma of the Vulva

To elucidate some of the factors influencing the outcome of the treatment of small vulvar carcinomas, the medical records and histological material from 117 patients with stage I lesions were reviewed [4]. FIGO stage I is defined as a tumour confined to the vulva, 2 cm or less in diameter, with nodes that are either not palpable, or are palpable but mobile and are not enlarged (i.e. not clinically suspicious of neoplasm).

Treatment methods in this series can be summarised as follows: 41 cases did not receive standard surgical treatment. Four were treated with local excision only, two with hemivulvectomy, and 35 with vulvectomy. Radical vulvectomy with groin (54) or groin and pelvic (22) lymphadenectomy was performed in a total of 76 cases. In 8 out of 41 cases (19.8%) not receiving radical surgical treatment, local and inguinal recurrences developed, while this occurred in only 12 out of 76 (15.8%) treated with radical vulvectomy and lymphadenectomy.

The relationship between depth of infiltration, vessel invasion, and recurrences was also studied. In 23 patients the tumour infiltrated less than 1 mm into the stroma, measured from the base of the epithelium from which the tumour developed. All these patients had an excellent prognosis and showed no invasion into vessels or lymph node metastases. No other relationship could be found between depth of infiltration up to 15 mm and occurrence of vessel invasion, recurrences and deaths. It must be admitted, however, that measurement of depth of infiltration was in most cases made from the surface of the tumour, which in retrospect was found to add several millimetres, in some cases, to the so-called depth of infiltration because of papular growth of the tumour.

The significance of vessel invasion in relation to lymph node metastases, recurrences in the groin and death from cancer was, however, quite clear. In the series of 76 cases which underwent lymphadenectomy, 6 out of 15 with vessel invasion had metastases compared with only 2 out of 61 without demonstrable vessel invasion. Of importance also is that in the series of 22 patients who underwent pelvic lymphadenectomy, none had metastases to this region. The importance of vessel invasion is also demonstrated by significantly more recurrences in the groin and deaths from cancer occurring in the group with, than in the group without, vessel invasion. In the total series of 117 cases, 5 out of 19 with vessel invasion developed groin metastases as compared with 2 out of 98 without vessel invasion. Moreover, 6 out of 19 with vessel invasion died from cancer, as compared with 4 out of 98 without vessel invasion.

Of great importance for a possible future treatment protocol is that of the total of eight cases with groin metastases, seven were located on the same side as the primary tumour. Bilateral metastases were found in only one case, and this patient had unquestionable invasion of tumour cells in capillary-like spaces, most probably lymphatic vessels.

Conclusion, Stage I

On the basis of this study, it is suggested that one should always have an excisional biopsy in stage I carcinoma of the vulva for a thorough histological examination of the depth of infiltration and especially to ascertain whether or not there are definite signs of involvement of endothelial-lined spaces.

It seems reasonable to recommend either hemivulvectomy, or in younger patients merely a wide excision as primary treatment, provided the tumour is unilateral and the infiltration is less than 1 mm.

If the infiltration exceeds 1 mm, hemivulvectomy should be combined with ipsilateral groin dissection (Fig. 25.2). If vessel invasion is found, it is necessary to perform bilateral groin lymphadenectomy (Fig. 25.3).

The above treatment protocol refers only to strictly unilateral lesions. If the tumour is located anteriorly near the midline, standard radical vulvectomy with

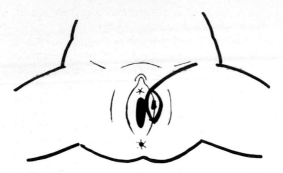

Fig. 25.2. Incision lines for hemivulvectomy with ipsilateral groin dissection.

bilateral lymphadenectomy is recommended, but it should be kept in mind that it is not necessary to remove a large part of the posterior vulva.

If the tumour is located posteriorly in the midline, vulvectomy with preservation of the clitoris and bilateral groin lymphadenectomy is recommended.

As to the definition of an entity called microcarcinoma of the vulva, our study seems to indicate that only tumours infiltrating less than 1 mm into the stroma should be allocated to such a group.

Stage II Carcinoma of the Vulva

Stage II carcinoma of the vulva is defined as a tumour confined to the vulva more than 2 cm in diameter without spread to the vagina, the urethra, the perineum or anus. Groin nodes may be palpable, but should not be clinically suspicious of neoplasms.

It is our experience that strictly unilateral stage II lesions seldom have bilateral metastases [5]. Bilateral metastases are usually only found when there are metastases to the ipsilateral groin nodes. Therefore, if the tumour is not larger than

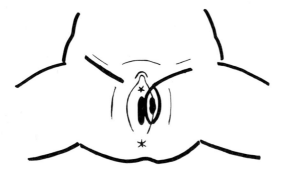

Fig. 25.3. Incision lines for bilateral groin lymphadenectomy.

3–4 cm in diameter, we agree with Morris [6] that it may in the first instance be justifiable to perform ipsilateral lymphadenectomy only. Contralateral metastases alone are extremely uncommon. In our own series this happened in only 1 of 53 cases with unilateral tumours. If a frozen section taken during operation does not reveal spread to the ipsilateral lymph nodes, contralateral groin dissection may be postponed until the final histological examination of the ipsilateral groin nodes is available. It should be emphasised that midline tumours in the clitoral region or the perineum always necessitate bilateral lymphadenectomy.

We would like to propose a final modification of the standard surgical treatment of stage II vulvar carcinoma, related to the question of preservation of the clitoris in women who have an active sexual life, irrespective of age. If a unilateral stage II lesion not more than 4 cm in diameter is located in the posterior half of the vulva, it may be justified to modify the incision line as indicated in Fig. 25.4. The clitoris, urethra and upper quarter of the vulva are preserved and a suprapubic flap is not fashioned.

It must be admitted that at present we do not have any series of stage II lesions treated in this way. However, there seems to be enough evidence to recommend that such a treatment protocol be set up in those institutions which have a long experience of the treatment of epidermoid carcinoma of the the vulva. Preservation of the clitoris should, however, not be attempted in stage II lesions located in the anterior half of the vulva. We base this on our experience that local recurrences represent a major problem in the treatment of vulvar carcinoma. Even if the primary tumour is removed with ample free margins, local recurrences were, in our own series, found in as many as 21.5% of 186 patients in stage II, III and IV treated by radical surgery. The recurrences usually appeared during the first two years of follow-up and were as a rule located at the site of the primary tumour. However, no fewer than 12 out of 40 local recurrences were detected more than 10 years after primary treatment. These recurrences were most probably new tumours developing in a potentially neoplastic field.

Our observation on the relatively high frequency of local recurrence is in agreement with the experience of other authors. It should lead to a wide and deep dissection of the tissues around the tumour, but should not necessarily involve a similar radical procedure on the contralateral side. This concept is illustrated by the asymmetrical incisions shown in Fig. 25.4.

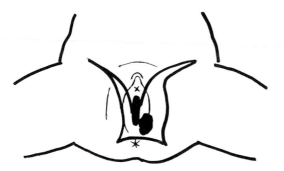

Fig. 25.4. Asymmetrical incisions for a lesion in the posterior half of the vulva.

References

1. Survival of cancer patients. Cases diagnosed in Norway 1953–75 (1981) The Cancer Registry of Norway, Oslo 3
2. Iversen T, Aalders JG, Christensen A, Kolstad P (1980) Squamous cell carcinoma of the vulva: A review of 424 patients, 1956–1974. Gynecol Oncol 9:271–279
3. Wharton JT, Gallager S, Rutledge FN (1974) Microinvasive carcinoma of the vulva. Am J Obstet Gynecol 118:159–162
4. Iversen T, Abeler V, Aalders J (1981) Individualized treatment of stage I carcinoma of the vulva. Obstet Gynecol 57:85–89
5. Iversen T (1981) Squamous cell carcinoma of the vulva. Localization of the primary tumor and lymph node metastases. Acta Obstet Gynaecol Scand 60:211–214
6. Morris J, McL (1977) A formula for selective lymphadenectomy. Its application to cancer of the vulva. Obstet Gynecol 50:152–158

26 · Management of Regional Lymph Nodes and Their Prognostic Influence on Vulvar Cancer*

N.F. Hacker, J.S Berek, L.D. Lagasse, R.S. Leuchter and J.G. Moore

Introduction

Within the past 5 years, two opposing points of view have been expressed regarding the extent of lymphadenectomy required for treatment of vulvar cancer. Krupp and Bohm suggested that optimum therapy required bilateral pelvic lymphadenectomy in addition to extended vulvectomy and bilateral inguinal lymphadenectomy [1]. On the other hand, Morris [2] advocated omitting the pelvic lymphadenectomy and the contralateral inguinal lymphadenectomy, provided that the primary tumour was unilateral and the ipsilateral inguinal-femoral nodes were negative.

Most authors suggest that invasive vulvar cancer should be treated by radical vulvectomy and bilateral groin dissection, reserving pelvic lymphadenectomy for patients with positive groin nodes [3–5]. However, Curry et al. [6] reported that none of their patients with fewer than four positive unilateral groin nodes had positive pelvic nodes, although two (8%) subsequently developed pelvic metastases. For patients with carcinoma of the clitoris or Bartholin's gland, pelvic lymphadenectomy has been considered part of the primary treatment [3,7,8]. Piver and Xynos [9] and Curry et al. [6], however, have shown recently that positive pelvic nodes are rare in the absence of inguinal-femoral nodal metastases in carcinoma of the clitoris. Leuchter et al. [10], reporting the present authors' data, demonstrated a similar experience for carcinoma of Bartholin's gland at the University of California, Los Angeles (UCLA).

* Reprinted with permission of the American College of Obstetricians and Gynecologists [Obstetrics and Gynecology (1983) 61:409]

In view of the controversy over the appropriate management of the groin and pelvic lymph nodes in patients with vulvar cancer, the authors have reviewed their experience with vulvar cancer in an effort to clarify this issue further and to assess the influence of positive lymph nodes on the prognosis of the disease.

Materials and Methods

From 1 July 1957 to 30 June 1978, 171 patients with primary invasive epidermoid carcinoma or adenocarcinoma of the vulva were seen at UCLA and City of Hope National Medical Center. One hundred and thirteen of these patients underwent radical vulvectomy and bilateral inguinal-femoral lymphadenectomy; in 98 patients, the groin dissections were performed through separate incisions [11], and 15 underwent an en bloc operation. Eighteen patients underwent a unilateral pelvic lymphadenectomy. All patients were followed for two years or longer, and 100 were followed for five years. Survival was calculated using a standard actuarial life-table method [12] corrected for death from intercurrent disease. Significance testing was performed by using the Mantel–Haenszel test [13].

Clinical Features

Of the 113 patients treated, 104 had squamous cell carcinoma, seven carcinoma of Bartholin's gland, and two adenocarcinoma underlying Paget's disease. Patients with melanoma or sarcoma were excluded. Distribution of the lesions was as follows: labium majus, 50; labium minus, 34; posterior fourchette, 8; perineum, 7; Bartholin's gland, 7; lateral vestibule, 4; and clitoris, 3. Nine of the labial lesions were bilateral. Fifty-six patients had stage I disease, 39 stage II, 16 stage III, and two stage IV. The mean age of the patients was 59 years, with a range of 30–84 years.

Thirty-one patients (27.4%) had positive inguinal-femoral lymph nodes. Twenty-eight of these had positive ipsilateral nodes and three had positive nodes bilaterally. No patient had positive contralateral nodes and negative ipsilateral nodes.

The incidence of positive inguinal-femoral nodes in relation to stage of disease and in comparison with lesion size for patients with squamous cell carcinoma is shown in Tables 26.1 and 26.2. Three or more positive groin nodes were present in no patient with stage I disease, in one (2.6%) with stage II, in six (37.5%) with stage III, and in two (100%) with stage IV disease.

Of the 31 patients with positive groin nodes, 15 underwent ipsilateral pelvic lymphadenectomy (Table 26.3). Of the 16 patients with one positive groin node, 10 received neither pelvic lymphadenectomy nor pelvic irradiation. Of the 6 patients with two positive unilateral groin nodes, only one had a pelvic lymphadenectomy, but two others received pelvic irradiation. Two of the three patients with three positive unilateral inguinal nodes had a unilateral pelvic

Table 26.1. Incidence of inguinal-femoral node metastases and stage of disease for epidermoid vulvar carcinoma

Stage	No.	Positive nodes	Percent
I	56	6	10.7
II	32	8	25.0
III	14	10	71.4
IV	2	2	100.00
Total	104	26	25

Table 26.2. Correlation of inguinal-femoral node metastases and lesion size for epidermoid vulvar carcinoma

Lesion size (cm)	No.	Positive nodes	Percent
<1	23	1	4.3
1–2	33	6	18.2
2–4	33	11	33.3
>4	15	8	53.3
Total	104	26	25.0

Table 26.3. Status of pelvic lymph nodes in relation to inguinal-femoral node metastases

Groin nodes	No.	Pelvic LND[a]	Pelvic RT[b]	Positive pelvic nodes	Pelvic recurrences
Negative	82	3	0	0	0
1 Positive	16	6	0	0	0
2 Positive	6	1	2	0	0
3 Positive	3	2	1	1	1
4 Positive	6	6	0	5	3
Total	113(31c)	18	3	6	4

[a] LND = lymph node dissection
[b] RT = radiation therapy
[c] Number of cases with positive inguinal-femoral nodes

lymphadenectomy: two positive obturator nodes were found in one; and no positive pelvic nodes were found in the other. The third patient with three positive unilateral groin nodes received pelvic irradiation, but subsequently developed a pelvic recurrence. All six patients with four of more positive inguinal nodes had a pelvic lymphadenectomy and five (83%) of these had positive pelvic nodes.

Results

The actuarial 5-year survival for patients with stage I cancer (corrected for death from intercurrent disease) was 98%, whereas it was 90% for stage II, 60% for stage III, and 0% for stage IV (Fig. 26.1). Crude actuarial 5-year survival for patients with negative lymph nodes was 85%, whereas for those with positive nodes it was 60% ($P < 0.01$). When corrected for death from intercurrent disease,

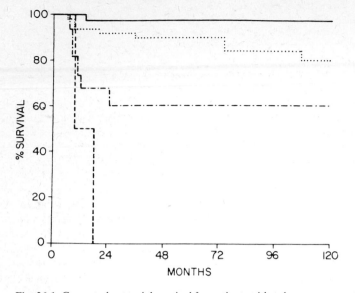

Fig. 26.1. Corrected actuarial survival for patients with vulvar cancer *vs* stage of disease. Solid line = stage I ($N = 56$); dotted line = stage II ($N = 39$); dot-dash line = stage III ($N = 16$), broken line = stage IV ($N = 2$).

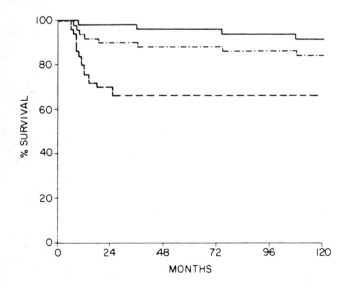

Fig. 26.2. Corrected actuarial survival for patients with vulvar cancer *vs* status of inguinal-femoral lymph nodes. Solid line = negative nodes ($N = 82$); broken line = positive nodes ($N = 31$); dot-dash line = all patients ($N = 113$), $P < .001$.

5-year survivals were 96% and 66%, respectively ($P < 0.001$) (Fig. 26.2). When analysed in relation to the number of positive lymph nodes, corrected actuarial 5-year survival was 94% for patients with one positive node, 80% for patients with two positive nodes, and 12% for patients with three or more positive nodes (Fig. 26.3). The influence of the number of positive nodes on survival is further emphasised when one examines patients with stage III disease. Of ten such patients with negative nodes or one positive node, none died of disease, whereas six of six stage III patients with three or more positive nodes died of disease.

Of the 82 patients with negative inguinal nodes, five (6%) died of disease. Of these, two developed pulmonary metastases, two developed recurrence in the vulva and groin, and one developed recurrence in the vulva and buttocks. None of these patients developed pelvic recurrences, including the 79 who did not have a pelvic node dissection or pelvic irradiation.

Of the 16 patients with one positive inguinal node, one died of disease with recurrences in the groin and vulva. This patient had bilateral vulvar lesions with squamous cell carcinoma, each measuring 3 cm in diameter. The only cancer-related death among the six patients with two positive inguinal nodes was from lung metastasis. This patient had a small (1 cm diameter) anaplastic carcinoma. Eight of the nine patients with three or more positive groin nodes died of disease. Site of recurrence in relation to nodal status is shown in Table 26.4.

No patient with tumour recurrence outside the vulva survived for any significant period of time. Four patients, however, developed an isolated vulvar recurrence and all were cured of their disease by re-excision with or without interstitial irradiation.

None of the six patients with metastases to pelvic lymph nodes demonstrated at pelvic lymphadenectomy survived.

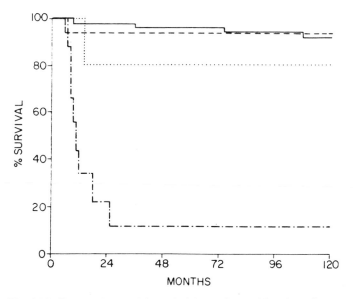

Fig. 26.3. Corrected actuarial survival for patients with vulvar cancer *vs* status of inguinal-femoral lymph nodes. Solid line = negative nodes ($N = 82$); broken line = one positive node ($N = 16$); dotted line = two positive nodes ($N = 6$); dot-dash line = three or more positive nodes ($N = 29$).

Table 26.4. Site of recurrence in relation to positive unilateral groin nodes

Nodal status	Vulva	Groin	Pelvis	Systemic
<3 positive	6/104 (5.8%)	3/104 (2.9%)	0/104 (0%)	4/104 (3.8%)
≥3 positive	3/9 (33%)	3/9 (33%)	4/9 (44%)	6/9 (66%)

In this series, pelvic lymphadenectomy increased operating time by about 45 min and increased mean blood loss by 250 ml (from 640 to 890 ml). The incidence of seromas also increased from 12% to 20% but there was no other increased morbidity and no associated operative mortality.

Discussion

Considerable controversy surrounds the extent of the lymph node dissection required for optimal treatment of vulvar carcinoma. For superficially invasive lesions, the issue concerns the need for groin dissection, while for frankly invasive lesions, most of the discussion concerns the indication for pelvic lymphadenectomy. Morris [2] has even questioned the need for contralateral groin dissection for patients with unilateral localised vulvar disease.

Green [14] and others [3,4,7] have reported no positive pelvic nodes in the absence of positive groin nodes. However, Green postulated that even if pelvic lymph nodes were histologically negative, submicroscopic disease might be present in up to 20% of cases, so the lymphadenectomy would by therapeutic for these patients. Curry et al. [6] reported that pelvic lymph nodes were positive in at least 8% of patients with fewer than four positive unilateral groin nodes; however, they were unable to determine the therapeutic value of pelvic lymphadenectomy because almost all patients in the series underwent this procedure.

The present data suggest that pelvic lymphadenectomy adds nothing to the cure of patients with histologically negative pelvic nodes. Seventy-nine patients with negative inguinal nodes did not undergo a pelvic lymphadenectomy, and the 5-year corrected actuarial survival for this group was 96%, the same as that for the entire group of 82 patients. Similarly, of the 16 patients with a single positive inguinal node, only six underwent pelvic lymphadenectomy and none underwent pelvic irradiation, yet there was only one death from cancer, and this was from recurrences in the groin and vulva. The corrected actuarial 5-year survival for this group was 94%.

Although some [1, 14] have reported no increased morbidity from the addition of pelvic lymphadenectomy to radical vulvectomy and bilateral groin dissection, others have not verified this [2,5]. Morris [2] reported that operative mortality could be reduced by 2% if pelvic lymphadenectomy were omitted, and Figge and Gaudenz [5] reported that major complications were twice as common in patients having pelvic lymphadenectomy than in those having groin dissection only. In the present series, only 18 pelvic lymphadenectomies were performed. There was a modest increase in blood loss and operating time in this group, but there was no operative mortality. The only difference in morbidity was a slight increase in the incidence of groin seromas.

No patient in the present series had positive pelvic nodes or developed a pelvic recurrence if there were one or two positive, unilateral inguinal nodes. Two of the three patients with three positive groin nodes had metastases to pelvic nodes, as did five of the six patients with four or more positive groin nodes. No patient with positive pelvic nodes was cured of disease.

Positive pelvic nodes were not found in the absence of palpably suspicious or fixed groin nodes. However, two of the seven patients (28.6%) with positive pelvic nodes or pelvic recurrence had primary vulvar lesions 2 cm or less in diameter. Histologically, both tumours were well differentiated large cell keratinising carcinomas, invasive to 6 and 10 mm, respectively. Thus, careful preoperative assessment of the groin nodes is one of the more accurate predictors of metastases to pelvic nodes. Size of the primary lesion appears less significant, although 71.4% of patients with metastases to pelvic nodes had primary lesions 3 cm or more in diameter.

These data, together with other reports [2,6], suggest that one should be selective in performing pelvic lymphadenectomy in patients with vulvar cancer. In view of the poor survival for patients with positive pelvic nodes and the increased operative morbidity and mortality associated with this procedure, the low incidence of positive pelvic nodes in patients with fewer than three positive unilateral groin nodes does not justify pelvic lymphadenectomy in this group of patients.

The advisability of omitting contralateral groin dissection in the presence of negative ipsilateral nodes remains debatable. Although no patient in the present and other series [2,14,16] had positive contralateral nodes in the absence of positive ipsilateral nodes, up to 15.3% of patients have been reported to have this pattern of tumour spread [1]. Because the exact site of the primary lesion is usually not stated, it is difficult to interpret reports of contralateral nodal disease in the absence of ipsilateral groin metastases. The present data suggest that it is extremely unlikely that a patient with a primary lesion on the midportion of the labium would develop contralateral node metastasis. However, in view of the poor prognosis for patients who develop subsequent metastases in an unresected groin [15] and the improved healing and relatively low morbidity associated with groin dissection through separate incisions [11], the authors are reluctant to omit contralateral groin dissection except for patients with unilateral superficially invasive lesions.

Survival correlated well with clinical stage, although on further analysis, it was shown that clinical stage correlated closely with the number of positive unilateral groin nodes. As an independent variable, the number of positive unilateral groin nodes correlated more closely with survival than did clinical stage.

The low incidence of local, regional and systemic tumour recurrences in patients with one or two positive unilateral groin nodes justifies the use of surgery alone in such patients. However, in view of the high incidence of pelvic and groin recurrence in patients with three or more positive unilateral groin nodes, strong consideration should be given to postoperative groin and pelvic irradiation for these patients. Studies of adjuvant chemotherapy are also warranted in view of the high incidence (66%) of systemic metastases of this group.

References

1. Krupp PJ, Bohm JW (1978) Lymph gland metastases in invasive squamous cell cancer of the vulva. Am J Obstet Gynecol 130:943–947

2. Morris JM (1977) A formula for selective lymphadenectomy. Obstet Gynecol 50:152–158
3. Morley GW (1976) Infiltrative carcinoma of the vulva: Results of surgical treatment. Am J Obstet Gynecol 124:874–884
4. Rutledge F, Smith JP, Franklin EW (1970) Carcinoma of the vulva. Am J Obstet Gynecol 106:1117–1126
5. Figge DC, Gaudenz R (1974) Invasive carcinoma of the vulva. Am J Obstet Gynecol 119:382–392
6. Curry SL, Wharton JT, Rutledge F (1980) Positive lymph nodes in vulvar squamous cell carcinoma. Gynecol Oncol 9:63–67
7. Benedet JL, Turko M, Fairey RN, et al. (1979) Squamous carcinoma of the vulva: Results of treatment 1938 to 1976. Am J Obstet Gynecol 134:201–206
8. Barclay DL, Collins CR, Macey AB (1964) Cancer of the Bartholin gland: A review and report of 8 cases. Obstet Gynecol 24:329–334
9. Piver MS, Xynos FP (1977) Pelvic lymphadenectomy in women with carcinoma of the clitoris. Obstet Gynecol 49:592–595
10. Leuchter RS, Hacker NF, Voet RL, et al. (1982) Primary carcinoma of Bartholin's gland: A report of 14 cases and review of the literature. Obstet Gynecol 60:361–368
11. Hacker NF, Leuchter RS, Berek JS, et al. (1981) Radical vulvectomy and bilateral inguinal lymphadenectomy through separate groin incisions. Obstet Gynecol 58:574–579
12. Kaplan EL, Meier O (1958) Nonparametric estimation from incomplete observations. JAMA 457:481–485
13. Mantel N (1966) Evaluation of survival and two new rank order statistics arising in its consideration. Cancer Chemother Rep 50:163–166
14. Green TH (1978) Carcinoma of the vulva. A reassessment. Obstet Gynecol 52:462–468
15. Iversen T, Aalders JG, Christensen A, et al. (1980) Squamous cell carcinoma of the vulva: A review of 424 patients, 1956–1974. Gynecol Oncol 9:271–279
16. Collins CG, Lee FYL, Roman-Lopez JJ (1971) Invasive carcinoma of the vulva with lymph node metastases. Am J Obstet Gynecol 109:446–452

27 · Myocutaneous Vulvo-vaginal Reconstruction

C. G. Lacey and C. P. Morrow

Introduction

As we reflect upon the vast scope of medical progress over the last quarter of a century or look even more specifically at surgical advances during this time, we find few techniques or innovations that provide tangible relief to a patient in terms of reduced pain and suffering or improved quality of life. In this regard the introduction and rapid growth of musculo-cutaneous flap surgery over the past decade has provided a humanitarian contribution to medicine of profound value. This is especially so in gynaecological oncology where the anatomical devastation from ultra-radical surgery or overzealous radiation therapy often leaves an agonising residuum in the form of an indolent or unhealing wound.

With great enthusiasm, therefore, gynaecological oncologists have implemented this new technique, and now commonly use myocutaneous flaps to reconstruct and renourish large denuded and devascularised vulvo-vaginal wounds. Because this technique has provided answers to problems that hereto obstinately defied solution it is not an exaggeration to say that it has been a major breakthrough in gynaecological surgery. This paper will briefly review the modern history of myocutaneous flaps and will illustrate the technical aspects of this procedure using the gracilis muscle as an example.

History

The contemporary history of myocutaneous reconstructive surgery often credits Owens [1] and Bakamjian [2] as the pioneers of this technique, but their reports were anteceded by Tansini's [3] more than half a century earlier, in which he described a new method of breast reconstruction using a latissimus dorsi compound flap (1896). Over the ensuing 50 years sporadic reports appeared in the literature describing many different muscle flaps used in a variety of anatomical locations. Garlock [4] in 1928 was one of the first to describe the gracilis muscle flap, which he used without the overlying skin to repair an intractable vesico-vaginal fistula. Orticochea [5] in 1972 first described the compound skin and muscle gracilis flap in his innovative paper on total reconstruction of the penis.

McGraw and Massey reported the first series of gracilis myocutaneous vaginal reconstruction operations following total pelvic exenteration [6]. Since their report, numerous others have appeared attesting to the utility and success of several different myocutaneous flaps for vulvo-vaginal reconstruction. Pertinent to the development of these grafts was the concept of the dominant vascular pedicle advanced by Vasconez [7] and the plastic surgery group in Atlanta, which provided a scientific explanation for the success of these techniques and showed the way for their widespread application.

Principles

The successful execution of a musclo-cutaneous flap depends upon the principle that some skeletal muscles and a predictable area of overlying skin and soft tissue are nourished by a dominant vascular pedicle. This pedicle provides an axis for isolation, elevation, and rotation of a myocutaneous unit to cover a near-by defect. The requirements for successful execution of the technique are: (a) relative proximity between the donor skin–muscle island (pedicle) and the recipient wound, (b) a patent and uninjured vascular pedicle, and (c) an expendable donor muscle that can be disconnected from its origin and/or insertion without appreciable loss of skeletal function. It is desirable, but not absolutely necessary, that the donor site has the potential for primary closure. This is not always possible in gynaecology, however, as in the case of the tensor fascia lata flap, where a split thickness skin graft may be necessary to cover the donor bed. Very recently, musculo-cutaneous units have been transferred to areas distant from the donor site by severing the dominant arterial pedicle and anastamosing it to another arteriole using microvascular techniques. These so-called free myocutaneous grafts have yet to be described in the gynaecological literature.

The most useful myocutaneous units for gynaecological purposes are the gracilis, tensor fascia lata, rectus femoris, and compound gluteus flap. The gracilis, because of its location, is the most versatile and commonly used and is selected here for detailed description.

Gross Anatomy

The gracilis muscle is located on the medial surface of the thigh. It originates from the lower portion of the symphysis pubis and the medial aspect of the inferior pubic ramus. It is a flat muscle that courses along the medial thigh where it consolidates distally into a tendon that passes behind the femoral condyle and inserts on to the medial surface of the upper tibia. It functions as an adductor of the thigh and flexor and medial rotator of the leg but it can be sacrificed without appreciable loss of skeletal function.

The muscle receives its dominant blood supply directly from a small, medial branch (1.2–1.5 mm) of the profunda femoris artery or from a branch of the medial circumflex femoral artery. This vessel courses between the adductor longus and adductor brevis to enter the deep aspect of the gracilis at a remarkably consistent location 7–9 cm from the pubic tubercle. This artery is accompanied by paired venae comitantes and a motor-sensory branch of the obturator nerve. There may be two or more distal contributions to the blood supply, but these are not critical to the survival of the muscle as long as the dominant vascular pedicle is preserved and uninjured. It is important to note that the skin overlying the distal one-third of the muscle receives its dominant blood supply from the sartorius muscle and therefore this skin should not be included in the gracilis flap.

Surgical Anatomy and Technique of the Operation

The patient is positioned in the support crutches with the thigh slightly flexed and adducted. The muscle is located by drawing a line obliquely downward from the pubic tubercle toward the insertion of the semi-tendonosus tendon on the upper medial surface of the tibia. This line reliably defines the anterior border of the gracilis muscle in the middle and distal portion of the thigh. An elliptical island is then outlined below this line with its widest point centred over the middle one-third of the gracilis muscle [8]. The length of the island is usually 20–25 cm and the width 6–8 cm, but the actual size will be dictated by the dimensions and proximity of the recipient wound. The distal ends of the ellipse meet at the junction of the middle and distal one-third of the gracilis muscle; this point of dissection is in close proximity to the intersection of the sartorius and gracilis muscles in the distal thigh. The proximal ends of the ellipse meet approximately 4–5 cm from the labio-crural fold. The island thus outlined is directly over the main body of the gracilis muscle from which it receives its dominant blood supply through fascial perforators. Once the flap has been accurately diagrammed, the operation may begin.

The muscle is located by incising the anterior border of the ellipse in the middle portion of the thigh. The incision is carried down through the fascia lata staying perpendicular to the surface to avoid undercutting and devascularising the skin periphery. Care must be taken here to avoid the greater saphenous vein, which travels parallel to the distal part of the incision which it may, in fact, traverse. Once beneath the fascia lata, a plane is identified between the adductor longus muscle anteriorly and the gracilis muscle behind. Using finger dissection behind the encompassing fascia, the muscle can be readily elevated distally and its posterior border identified. The posterior incision is generally made along the posterior border of the gracilis muscle belly, but in contrast to the anterior skin incision, which must closely follow the anterior muscle border, an additional 1–2 cm of skin may be reliably included posteriorly. The muscle is divided above the knee at the junction of its middle and distal one-third after first securing the fascia to the muscle with heavy absorbable sutures proximal and distal to the point of transection. The dissection is then carried cephalad and any minor vascular pedicles beneath the muscle may be sacrificed. The dominant vascular pedicle must be positively identified 7–9 cm from the pubic tubercle exiting between the adductor longus and adductor brevis muscles (Fig. 27.1). Further sharp dissection above this dominant pedicle may be necessary to mobilise the flap sufficiently, particularly if its ultimate destination is the vagina.

If the flap is used for vaginal reconstruction, a generous subcutaneous tunnel is developed beneath the skin bridge from the vaginal defect to the proximal end of the thigh incision. (Fig. 27.2) For perineal or vaginal reconstruction, the flaps are rotated posteriorly, the left clockwise and the right counterclockwise. After rotating the flaps through the subcutaneous skin bridge on to the perineum, they are gently supported while being sutured in place. A 'neovagina' is created by suturing the skin edges of the graft with a running absorbable suture to form a pouch (Fig. 27.3). This new vagina is then rotated posteriorly into the vaginal defect. The apex is sutured to the sacral fascia by an abdominal team and the perineal skin edges are approximated to the vulvar skin with an absorbable suture. The healed introitus is depicted in Fig. 27.4.

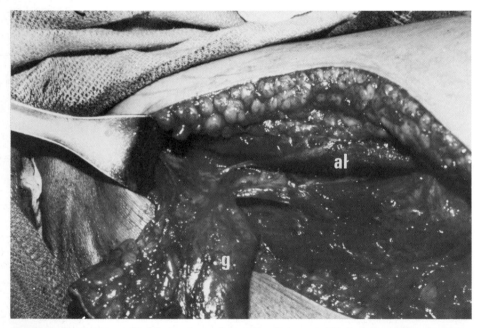

Fig. 27.1. Dominant gracilis (g) vascular pedicle exiting between adductor longus (al) and adductor brevis muscles.

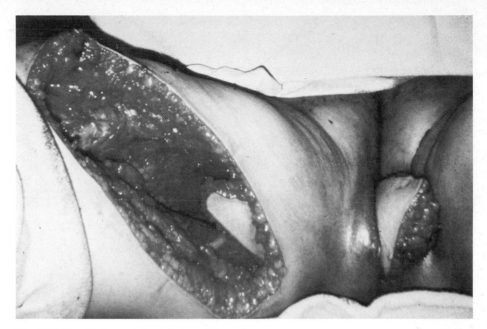

Fig. 27.2. Gracilis flap rotated into tunnel to perineum.

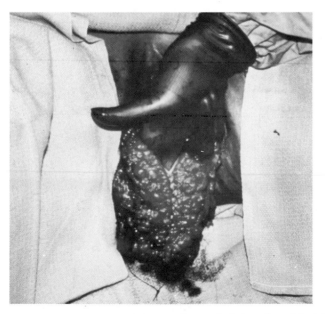

Fig. 27.3. Neovagina which is rotated posteriorly into the pelvic defect.

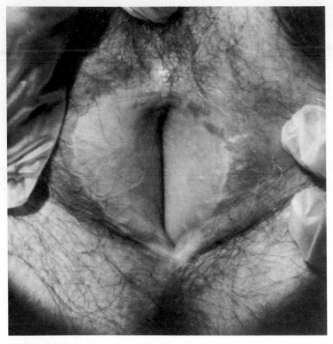

Fig. 27.4. Healed introitus. The interface between vulva and transferred skin is easily recognised.

For large groin defects, the operation is designed so that the anterior thigh incision intersects the inferior groin incision. The two wounds are thus joined and the graft may be rotated directly into the defect (Fig. 27.5). In this instance, the flaps are rotated anteriorly, the left counterclockwise and the right clockwise.

The thigh wound is closed over a suction drain with four or five number one or two synthetic monofilament full thickness retention sutures, which remain untied until the skin is approximated with a running nylon suture or staples. The retention sutures are tied over a gauze bolster (Fig. 27.6). Forceful manual approximation of the thigh wound by the assistant is usually required to secure closure. The suction drain may be removed in 48 h if drainage is minimal, i.e. less than 25 cc per 24 h. The bolster dressing and retention sutures are removed after 5 days.

There are certain technical aspects of the procedure which bear emphasis. When the leg is supported in the operating crutches, the thigh is suspended between the operating table which supports the torso, and the crutch which supports the calf. In this position, the medial strap muscles and soft tissue of the thigh hang toward the floor and the tendency is to make the anterior incision too far forward. When there is doubt about the location of the gracilis muscle, a 2–3 cm vertical incision in the distal thigh may be used to locate the gracilis tendon. The gracilis, which is composed of muscle and tendon, can be recognised from the sartorius, which is all muscle, and the semi-membranosus, which is all tendon. Traction on the gracilis tendon will elevate the muscle and appropriate overlying skin. The skin and subcutaneous incision must be perpendicular to the fascia along its entire length to avoid undercutting the skin, and as mentioned

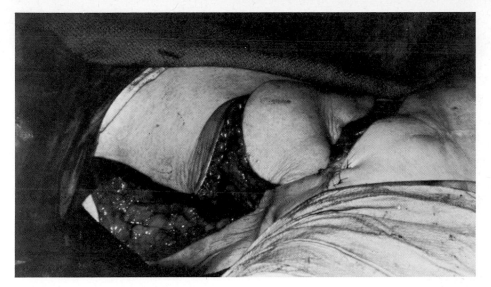

Fig. 27.5. Gracilis flap rotated directly into a large groin defect.

previously, caution is necessary during the distal anterior skin incision to avoid the greater saphenous vein, which traverses a course parallel and in close proximity to the anterior incision. Once the flap is elevated the skin and subcutaneous tissue must be kept in close apposition to the the fascia and muscle at all times. We achieve this by temporarily suturing the skin to the fascia lata at 5–6 cm intervals around the graft. Perhaps most importantly, the dominant vascular pedicle must

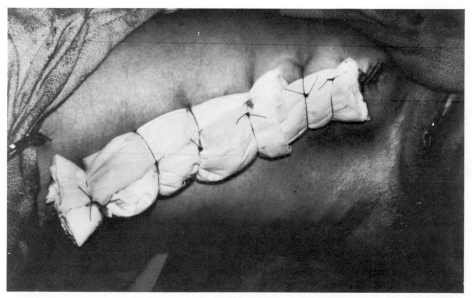

Fig. 27.6. Bolster dressing with suction drain exiting above the distal end.

be positively identified and care taken to prevent tension, torsion, or compression of this vital link to survival of the unit. Finally the graft must be sutured into place without tension. Persistent skin appendages ('dog ears') at the ends of the thigh incision frequently provide the only bothersome sequelae and may be excised at the time the leg wounds are closed.

Uses, Advantages and Disadvantages and Complications

The gracilis flap is useful for large vulvo-vaginal defects, but it can be excessively bulky depending upon the amount of subcutaneous tissue in the leg and should not be used when bulk is unnecessary or undesirable. It is ideal for large vaginal or inguinal radiation ulcers, where it provides both cover and new blood supply, and for vaginal reconstruction following total pelvic exenteration, where it additionally provides bulk to fill the large pelvic void. The major disadvantage of its use in this situation is a fairly consistent loss of tactile sensation which reduces its effectiveness as a sexual organ. The muscle has also been used alone for repair of recurrent vesico-vaginal or recto-vaginal fistulae. It offers the advantage of close proximity to the perineum and vagina, and has a long arc of rotation. Furthermore, the success of the flap is reasonably predictable when the anatomical and technical requirements of the operation are observed. The tensor fascia lata flap from the lateral thigh or the rectus femoris flap from the anterior thigh may offer advantages over the gracilis for some groin, pubic or perineal defects depending upon their size and location. The posterior thigh flap is technically more complicated than the gracilis but may provide better sensation which may make it more attractive for vaginal reconstruction.

Complete or partial flap loss can occur and this is especially so along the anterior distal margin of the gracilis. This can be avoided by good surgical technique and by confining the skin margins to the anatomical limits of the gracilis muscle. Intravenous fluorescein (10–15 mg/kg) has been recommended by some as a simple immediate test for flap viability in the operating room. Nevertheless, when partial or complete necrosis does occur, timely debridement is necessary to avoid the septic consequences which sometimes ensue from such a reservoir of bacterial growth and putrefaction. Often, when only the skin and subcutaneous tissue infarct, the surviving muscle may provide sufficient new blood supply to heal the wound. It is, therefore, sometimes necessary to stage the debridement to avoid resection of viable tissue.

Fundamentally, the complications are all vascular in origin and consequently careful design and technical diligence are the elements of success. Once the flap is elevated and the dominant pedicle identified and isolated, every effort must be expended to prevent vascular compromise. Shearing forces on the small perforators between the fascia and subcutaneous tissue must be prevented by systematically suturing the skin to the fascia lata as the flap is elevated. If the flap is tunnelled the surgeon must provide an extra measure of room in anticipation of the venous and lymphatic swelling which inevitably accompany this procedure. Vascular thrombosis due to torsion or tension is avoided by supporting the graft at all times. These self evident rules of common sense are uniformly recognised by experienced surgeons as the margin between success and failure.

References

1. Owens NA (1955) A compound neck pedicle designed for the repair of massive facial defects: formation, development, and application. Plast Reconstr Surg 15:369–389
2. Bekamjian MY (1963) A technique for primary reconstruction of the palate after radical maxillectomy for cancer. Plast Reconstr Surg 31:103–117
3. Tansini I (1896) Nuovo processo per l'amputazione della mammaella per cancre. La Reforma Medica 12:3–8
4. Garlock JH (1928) The cure of an intractable vesico-vaginal fistula by the use of a pedicled muscle flap. Surg Gynecol Obstet 47:255–260
5. Orticochea M (1972) A new method of total reconstruction of the penis. Br J Plast Surg 25:347–399
6. McCraw JB, Massey FM (1976) Vaginal reconstruction with gracilis myocutaneous flaps. Plast Reconstr Surg 58:176–183
7. McCraw JB. Vasconez LO (1980) The recent history of myocutaneous flaps. In: Clinics in Plastic Surgery, vol 7, pp 3–9
8. Morrow CP, Lacey CG, Lucas WE (1979) Reconstructive surgery in gynecologic cancer employing the gracilis myocutaneous pedicle graft. Gynecol Oncol 7:176–187

Breast

28 · Contact X-ray Microscopy of the Breast

R.Ll. Davies, J.K. Pye and I.H. Gravelle

Introduction

The technique of contact X-ray microscopy is a means of studying the microstructure of various tissues. In particular, it enables comparison of cellular densities and plays a role in the interpretation of mammographic patterns. The technique of X-ray microscopy has been available for many years but has been little used in the study of breast tissue [1,2]. The advantages offered by X-ray microscopy in the study of breast disease are due to the wavelengths of X-rays, which are approximately 1000 times shorter than those of visible light. This results in increased penetration and higher resolving power, enabling sections of biological tissue several hundred microns thick to be examined.

John Wolfe, a radiologist from Detroit, maintains that the mammographic appearance of breast parenchyma provides a method of predicting the risk for development of breast cancer [3]. He described four main groups shown in Fig. 28.1:

N1. Parenchyma composed primarily of fat and no ducts visible (low risk group).

P1. Parenchyma mainly fat, but prominent ducts present in the anterior portion of the breast up to a quarter of its volume (low risk group).

P2. More severe involvement noted, with a prominent duct pattern occupying more than a quarter of the volume of the breast (high risk group).

DY. Severe involvement, with dysplasia which often obscures an underlying prominent duct pattern (highest risk group).

Although there has been controversy about the interpretation of these findings, Wolfe has calculated that patients with a DY pattern have a 27 times increased risk of future breast cancer development compared with those having an N1

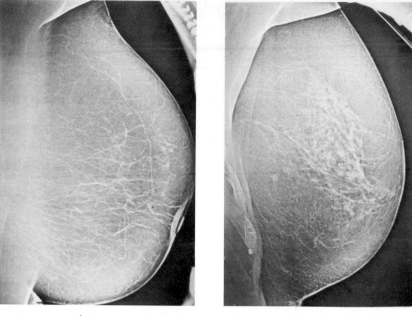

NI   PI

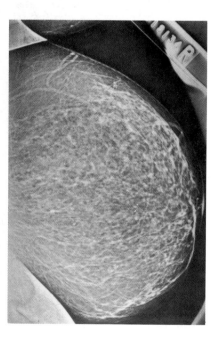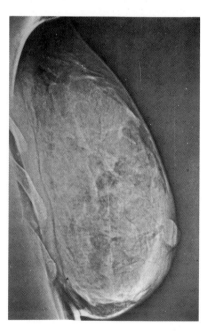

P2   DY

Fig. 28.1. Example of parenchymal patterns described by Wolfe.

pattern. We have therefore undertaken a study of the histological basis for the patterns of densities seen on mammograms.

Materials and Method

Breast tissue from open biopsy or mastectomy specimens, as in our research programme, may be used. Mastectomy specimens were obtained from patients having mastectomy for carcinoma. Prior to surgery, these patients had a xeromammogram that was coded according to Wolfe's criteria. The mastectomy specimens were delivered to the Pathology Department unfixed and were deep frozen at 70 °C for 1–1.5 h, depending on size. The breast was then sliced into 2 mm thick slices from medial to lateral. Slices through the nipple, medial, and lateral aspects of the breast were then selected and these slices were radiographed using a Faxitron. Areas of density on the radiographs of the slices were marked deep to the nipple, in the lower inner quadrant, and the upper outer quadrant. The equivalent areas were excised from the slices as blocks of tissue 0.75 × 0.75 × 0.2 cm. A 50 μm thick section was taken from each block and was further studied by X-ray microscopy. The cut sections were placed in formalin or distilled water and floated onto a 4 μm thick Mylar membrane stretched over a metal ring, as shown in Fig. 28.2. Excess fluid was removed with a micropipette, and the specimen was freeze dried and placed on a holder in contact with a disc of high

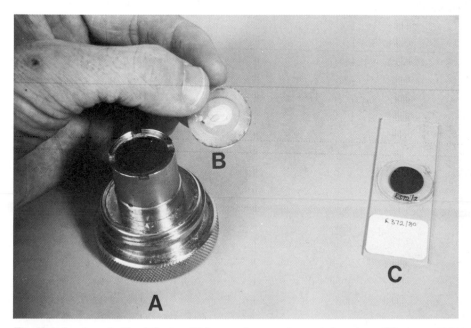

Fig. 28.2. Specimen holder (*A*); ring, Mylar membrane and mounted specimen (*B*); mounted microradiograph (*C*).

resolution film. The holder, with specimen and film, was mounted into the microradiography unit, which produces low-energy X-rays with wavelengths in the range of 0.83 to 0.18 nm (Softex CMR, Hosoda, Japan). The X-ray microscopic factors used were 2.5 kV, 3.0 mA for 5 min exposure onto Kodak high resolution film type S0343. Following this, the disc of exposed film was developed in the usual manner. In order to obtain a direct comparison with histological features the same piece of tissue, having been subjected to X-ray microscopy, was then stained with haematoxylin and eosin. The developed microradiograph and the stained tissue were mounted adjacently on the same microscope slide and viewed under a light microscope.

Examples of Microradiographs

Some of the microradiographs of aspects of normal breast tissue obtained in this study are illustrated in Figs. 28.3–28.6. Figure 28.3 shows the microradiograph of a section of breast tissue 50 μm thick. The appearances are as for conventional radiographs, with white areas representing radiodense structures and dark areas transradiant structures. It should be noted that no radio-opaque contrast media or staining techniques have been used and these differences are attributable to the varying densities of the cellular structures. In this figure two nipple ducts are seen in transverse section with stroma surrounding them. Figure 28.4 is from a section

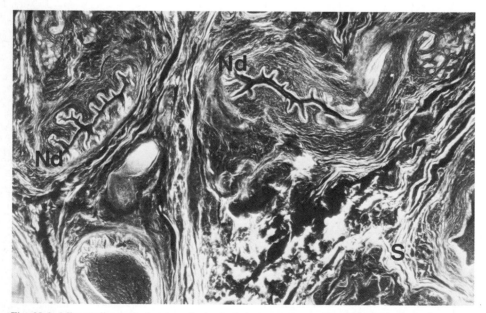

Fig. 28.3. Microradiograph showing nipple ducts in transverse section *Nd*, nipple duct; *S*, stroma. (×95).

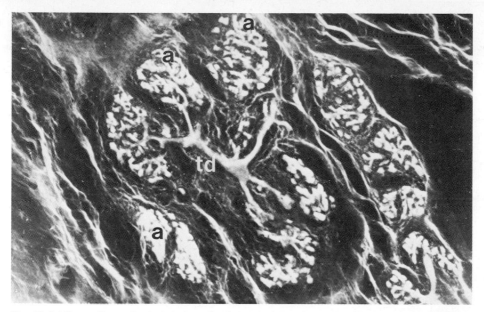

Fig. 28.4. Microradiograph of a lobular unit *td*, terminal ductule; *a*, alveoli of the lobule. (×95).

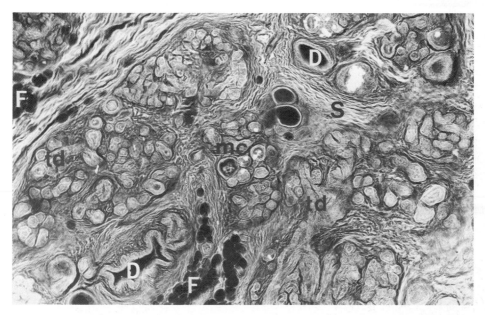

Fig. 28.5. Microradiograph of breast structure; *D*, duct; *td*, terminal ductule; *a*, alveoli of the lobule; *S*, stroma; *F*, fat; *mc*, microcalcification. (×95).

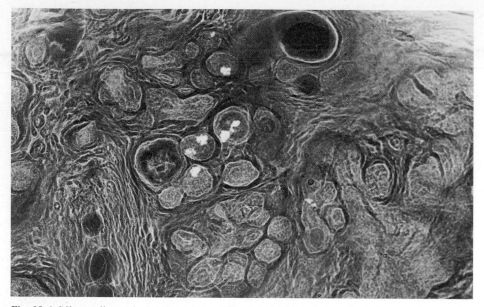

Fig. 28.6. Microradiograph showing microcalcification at higher power. (×190).

50 μm thick and shows a lobular unit with the terminal ductules and alveoli of the lobules.

Figure 28.5 demonstrates most of the features that can be observed on microradiographs of breast tissue. The 50 μm thick section shows the following features. A duct is seen in transverse sections and adjacent lobules are seen; one of these contains some microcalcification. The background stroma is clearly shown in collagenous strands and fat cells are also present. The lobule containing the microcalcification is seen at higher power in Fig. 28.6 and demonstrates the amorphous character of this type of calcification. Calcification appears to form in, or close to, ductules or lobules as small particles approximately 1 μm in diameter, and may coalesce to form larger deposits.

Summary

Contact X-ray microscopy has several advantages over conventional histological and radiological methods of correlation. The main advantage of this technique is that it permits the use of thicker specimens than conventionally used for histology. It is well known that adjacent sections of breast tissue can vary widely when 5 μm thick sections are being used. 50 μm thick sections enable the overall structure of a lobule or duct system to be easily discerned with virtually no overlap of structures. Standard histology allows various elements of epithelial atypia to be identified but the overall architecture cannot be fully appreciated. Contact X-ray microscopy is ideally suited to this tissue thickness and provides details of the relative densities of each breast component: this cannot be shown using standard radiological techniques.

In this study X-ray microscopy has proved to be an invaluable tool for assessment of the microdensity of breast structures, i.e. ducts, lobules, stroma and fat. A recent addition to this technique is the use of a reference wedge incorporated into each microradiograph as a standard for direct comparison between different microradiographs. This is a recent development but will allow analysis of microscopic breast density in relation to Wolfe's grades. This may provide a means of identifying a mechanism by which cancer risk can be predicted on the basis of mammographic parenchymal patterns. In addition, one of the earliest signs of underlying breast pathology on mammography is the presence of microcalcification. This is easily demonstrated using contact X-ray microscopy and may well have an application in this area.

A further advantage of this technique is that it brings together radiologists, surgeons and pathologists, providing a multidisciplinary approach to the difficult field of breast disease.

References

1. Barth V (1977) Die Feinstruktur der Brustdruse im Röntgenbild. Thieme, Stuttgart
2. Davies RLl (1983) Contact microradiography in bio-medical research. MSc thesis, University of Wales
3. Wolfe JN (1976) Risk for breast cancer development by mammographic parenchymal patterns. Cancer 37:2486–2492
4. Wolfe JN, Albert S, Belle S, Salane M (1982) Breast parenchymal pattern: Analysis of 332 incident breast carcinomas. AJR 138:113–118

Subject Index